Nigel Barker's

BEAUTY EQUATION

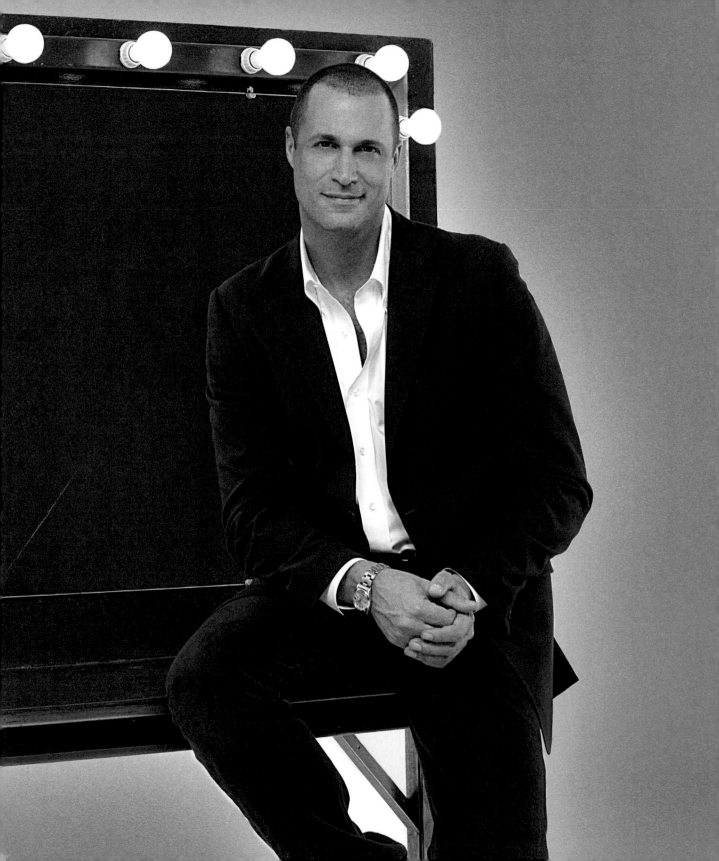

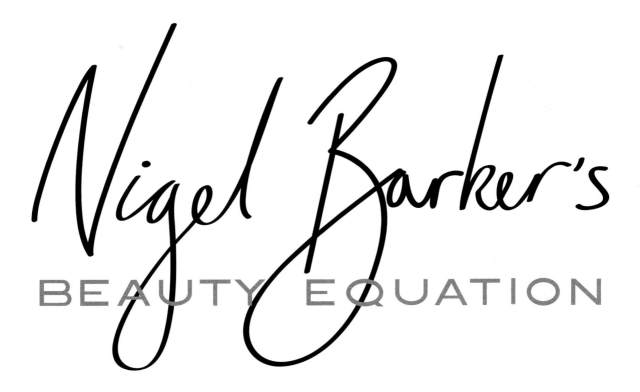

Nigel Barker's BEAUTY EQUATION

REVEALING A BETTER AND MORE BEAUTIFUL YOU

ABRAMS IMAGE, NEW YORK

My life, as well as this book, is dedicated to my beautiful wife, Crissy,
and our wondrous children, Jack and Jasmine.
Through my wife I found inner peace,
and through my children I discovered the future.

Contents

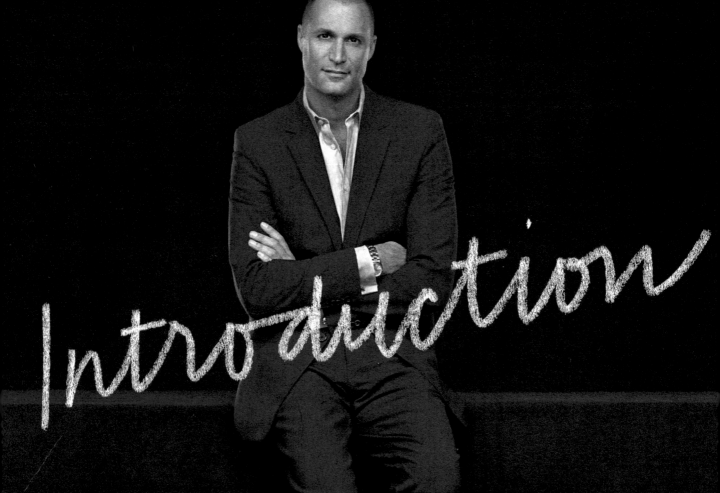

Introduction

you + allure + confidence + compassion
spontaneity + radiance + health +
honesty + charm + energy ÷ humor =

beauty

Introduction: *beauty*

WHAT IS BEAUTY, where does it stem from, and how do we obtain it? These are eternal questions, long pondered by queens and princesses, mothers and daughters, and experts and scholars alike.

I have been in the beauty business for the best part of twenty years, both in front of and behind the lens. But it was only when I became a dedicated photographer, charged with capturing the essence of beauty in everything I train my lens on, that it truly dawned on me what the secret to real beauty is. Until then, I, like most people, had been suckered into upholding modern society's notion of beauty. But the truth is that what most of us call beautiful is merely the current cultural definition of pretty: strong cheekbones, a slender body type, vibrant hair color. These are all without a doubt outer measurements of certain levels of attractiveness. But we all know people who are pretty but who are not beautiful. And we also know people who are not what would be described as classically pretty but who are undeniably beautiful. You've heard it said a million times before: Beauty comes from within. So what does that mean? How can you harness your own beauty? How can you exude it in a photograph and, even more importantly, in your everyday life?

The *Beauty Equation* sets out to slam shut Pandora's makeup box by unleashing ten of the essential qualities that add up to inner beauty. Unveil these and I guarantee you will find yourself uncovering your outer beauty as well.

THE ART BEHIND
THE SCIENCE OF BEAUTY

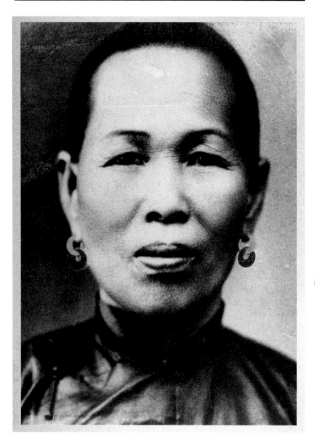

Crissy Barker's great-great-grandmother, Mrs. Chin

Defining beauty has been a holy grail for countless cultures throughout time, each putting their own spin on the notion of beauty, often with dreadful and even life-threatening consequences.

In ancient China (and continuing up until the past century), there was something in vogue called the lotus foot, achieved by breaking a young woman's toes and binding them under her feet to make the feet look as small as possible. Small feet, it was widely thought, looked attractive, demure, and modest. Well, it certainly was humbling—but for all the wrong reasons. My wife's great-great-grandmother had her feet bound and it caused her excruciating pain throughout her life.

Ancient Egyptians, Romans, and Persians loved big, sparkling eyes, and to achieve the look, applied black makeup laced with a heavy metal that caused eye injury and facial deformations.

In England during the time of Queen Elizabeth, big foreheads were all the rage (or should I say "rash"?). Women would actually pluck the hair out of the front of their head to create the look. And as if that wasn't bad enough, the Elizabethan ladies liked to cover their skin in an early form of foundation that was heavily lead based, often resulting in disfiguring scars and a lack of bowel control. How attractive!

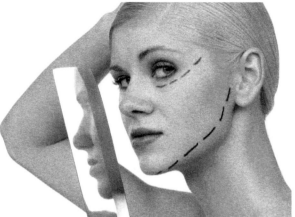

America's Next Top Model (ANTM) contestant Rebecca Epley

Today, of course, not only do we retouch our exteriors with a cacophony of makeup routines, but we go under the knife and actually cut away parts we don't like and add bits we do. That's not to say reconstructive surgery can't be very beneficial—I'm sure many of those Elizabethan chicks would have loved a face-lift after the makeup routine they were using.

While these shenanigans in the name of vanity have provoked women, regardless of era, to self-doubt and self-mutilate, they have also, ironically, stimulated philosophers and other great minds to ponder: What is beauty and how can it be acquired? The ancient Chinese were simultaneously binding feet, literally crippling their daughters, and putting out philosophy that said true beauty came from a good reputation, good behavior, talent, and longevity. The great Socrates, who pondered all realms of the universe, also delved into the beauty debate, suggesting in his accounts that a person who might appear attractive on the outside is not truly so if he has evil intentions—before going on to dismiss all expressions of physical beauty as untrustworthy.

The Pythagoreans had a theory—still in discussion today, believe it or not—called the golden section, that essentially says you can measure beauty by a set of mathematical proportions. Demonstrated by famous artworks like Leonardo's *Mona Lisa* and *Vitruvian Man* and Michelangelo's *David*, it's a rigid formula for attractiveness that suggests that certain measurable elements—say, the distance between your cheekbones, or the length and breadth of your nose, or the size of your eyes compared with the depth of your brow—can make you more physically attractive. But doesn't that point to an averageness that is boring and uninspiring? After all, we are not frozen statues—we are living, breathing people! Sure, you can find symmetry on someone's face when it's static, but get them to smile, frown, or just plain move and that symmetry changes in accordance with, for example, how confident they are at smiling. What someone looks like in motion— their body language—plays a big role in whether we find that someone attractive.

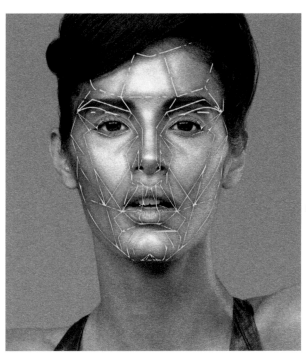

True beauty comes from the way you smile and sound and shimmy. We are made to be unique; our imperfections make us special. Even in sunlight, surely the perfect example of spontaneity, power, energy, and life, there is asymmetry—bursts, movement, waves.

Modern beauty concepts—glorifying superyoung, unhealthily skinny models with Photoshopped, unobtainably flawless skin—are not only misguiding, but they are no more a measure of true beauty, in my opinion, than plucked foreheads and tiny clubfeet. Real beauty—and this comes from years of searching for it and trying to photograph it—exists in everyone.

I'd argue that the true measure of beauty is, in fact, the measure of the emotion it stimulates. In other words, maybe you can't help but judge yourself against the current model physique—some girl five feet ten inches tall, weighing in at 115 pounds, with perfect teeth, who can glide down a runway as if she first learned to walk with six-inch heels on. Maybe, in your initial awe, you find yourself wishing you were slimmer or taller or more curvaceous than you are. But however outwardly attractive she may be, I promise you that what has attracted you to her is directly connected to whether she is confident, compassionate, honest, charming, or energetic. A model might have the looks to strut her stuff down a catwalk, but only when outer beauty is paired with other attributes of inner beauty does a woman resonate as truly gorgeous.

We all know the saying "The eyes are the windows to the soul," but, going further, they are also the windows to the heart and the mind, not to mention the very focus of almost every great photograph and conversation. I'm here to encourage your uniqueness, the way you move and present yourself, the way you bear witness to the

"Beauty is not based on just our bone structure. It is something that comes from within; it is something that we embody."

—*ANTM* winner Jaslene Gonzalez, masked by the dimensions of the "golden section" life you have led—your story—so that it can all resonate through your eyes and your smile in a way that is a thousand times more powerful than you have so far allowed yourself to believe. But you will have to learn how to let your true self come out through every inch of your body.

I have seen a room filled with model types where everybody's attention was fixed on some beautiful spirit, far from model perfection, but oozing with talent, charm, grace, and glamour. So maybe you think you don't have perfect skin, a great smile, or a swimsuit body—but what you do have, or could have, is far more alluring, sexy, timeless, and powerful. It's called *you*.

"When I find someone beautiful, it is more than a science. It is about presence and who you are."

—*ANTM* contestant
April Wilkner, pictured as the *Vitruvian (Wo-)Man*

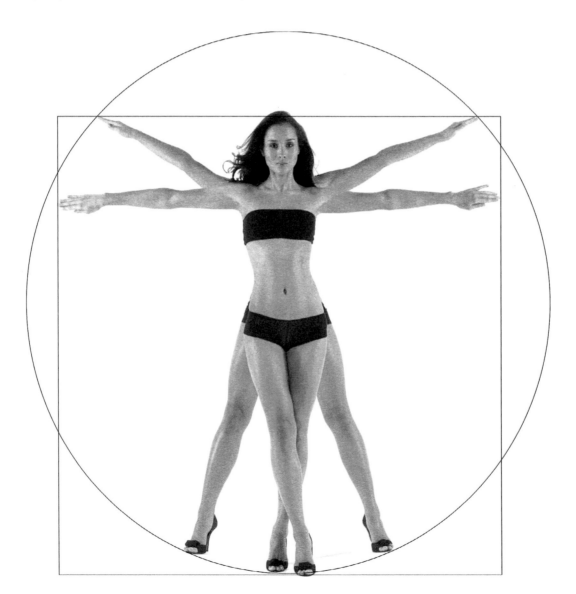

HOW TO USE THIS BOOK

This is your workbook and the ultimate project is a better and more beautiful you. By following the "teaches" and challenges laid out in the pages ahead, you will be empowered to discover your own Beauty Equation.

In each chapter, we will discuss an attribute of the Beauty Equation and I will share my knowledge and know-how with you. Working in the fashion industry, I have heard just about every rationale and excuse as to why someone is or isn't beautiful. I am going to tell you what I think beauty is, but I am also going to ask you to discover your own true beauty, through your own eyes.

I am inviting you to come with me on a journey of self-evaluation. Drawing on my experiences working with everybody from fashion-industry divas to single mothers in war-torn countries, I hope to work with you to show you how to shine from within. I can't promise you that it will be easy, because even with all my years of being surrounded by it, I am still sometimes surprised at the places real beauty hides.

Here is our secret weapon: The camera never lies. So by rising to the challenge of taking a series of self-portraits and doing other instructive photo assignments, confronting some demons, and answering a number of simple, pointed questions, we can work together to reveal the inner you in all your glory. Together, we are going to use the camera to dispel popular myths—like the idea that beauty is only skin-deep. "Pretty" may be skin-deep. Beauty, however, is an elusive combination. It's your inner essence combined with what people see, physically, when they look at you. When the equation all comes together, beauty seems effortless, but I'm here to tell you that "effortless beauty" requires a lot of work.

As a photographer, I work in many areas of the business—in fashion, shooting young models; in portraiture, shooting actors, musicians, and politicians; and in my favorite medium, looking for beauty in real-life situations, like in the poorest neighborhoods of Haiti, AIDS clinics in Tanzania, or the ice floes of eastern Canada. It's my job to nurture, coax, or seduce the beauty from my subject, whoever and wherever they may be. I often instruct my subjects to try and forget about the camera and engage them in conversation while shooting them so that I can capture those in-between moments. You've seen them in real life—real moments of beauty; occasions when you look across a room and see someone laughing, just being themselves, and in that moment, simply because of, say, the way they move, you fall for them. Capture that moment on camera and you have captured magic.

"Hang on, Nigel," you say. "I never take a good picture." Well, get ready, because you're going to take some now! But first, you may have to change your perception of what it means to look, feel, and be beautiful.

GETTING STARTED

I am about to take you through a series of teaches and challenges that I use and practice every day on my quest to capture beauty.

I know it sounds like I'm saying that as long as you're beautiful inside, you'll look beautiful on the outside too; and though I personally think that could be true, this book contains many physical challenges you'll need to rise to. The way you look after yourself, often from the inside, can affect your exterior beauty. For example, being proud will help you stand up straight and appear more confident. Living a more compassionate life will help you see beauty where before you thought there was none. Throughout the *Beauty Equation*, we will break down each area of your self-presentation so that you can be your most beautiful self, inside and out. I'll give you some simple advice on makeup application, how less is often more and how sometimes a little bit more is OK! And don't forget that another part of the equation is taking care of yourself through health and fitness.

Through this book and the teaches and challenges that it contains, you will create a working portfolio/diary of all the facets of your inner beauty, culminating in "You Be the Judge," where the various fractions all get added together to reveal your personal Beauty Equation.

You are going to make a portfolio of photos, words, and inspiration detailing, visually and verbally, how truly beautiful you are and can be. Just like the dynamic portfolio of a top model, filled with a full range of their best shots, your portfolio will highlight your best attributes and show the true you.

Think of the photos you will be taking as your reflections, saved for you to examine. By actually exuding your emotions and feelings through your eyes, and following the various challenges, you will be able to see your heart and soul begin to shine right out of those photographs. And then, keeping all of that in mind, you will know what to do when you want to look, feel, and be beautiful anyplace you go.

WHAT YOU NEED TO DO FIRST

Arm yourself with a camera. You can use pretty much any type of camera, as long as you can take pictures and video with it (see my chapter on photo tips for guidance on page 196). And you can either print out your photos and paste them into a scrapbook (keeping your video challenges on tape, DVD, or your computer desktop), or you can go completely digital, using the online resource we've created for you. If the latter is the way you want to go, check out the following:

www.beautyequation.com

This is the Web address for the Beauty Equation, where I encourage you to create your own profile and keep track of your own progress. Every challenge will tell you exactly how to name your photos and videos. If you follow the easy instructions provided on the Web site, posting will be a snap.

Remember, just like with an actual notebook at home, you can opt to let others view your portfolio or keep it for your eyes only. On the Web site, you will be able to read additional quotes from me and other noteworthy folks in the book and see firsthand what your peers have to say. I'll be a constant presence, not there to judge you, but rather to give you encouragement and a few words of advice.

All that being said, experiment and have fun, and please don't get too worried about the photo-taking elements of the book. It doesn't make a bit of difference how handy you are with a camera. What matters most is using the challenges to help you concentrate on being the best you.

YOUR FIRST CHALLENGE

Take a couple of simple head shots, and upload them as your starting photographs for your personal portfolio. If you are using www.beautyequation.com, log in and create your profile to upload your images. These photos will act as a point of reference from here on out.

Now, let's get started with the Beauty Equation!

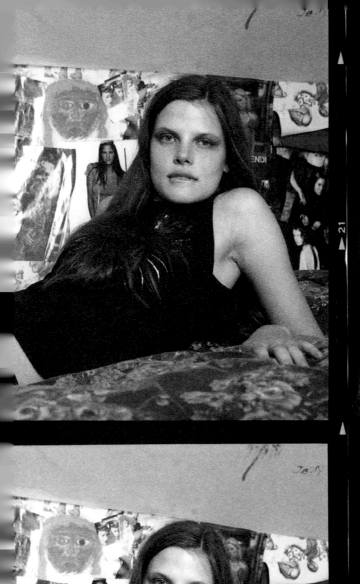
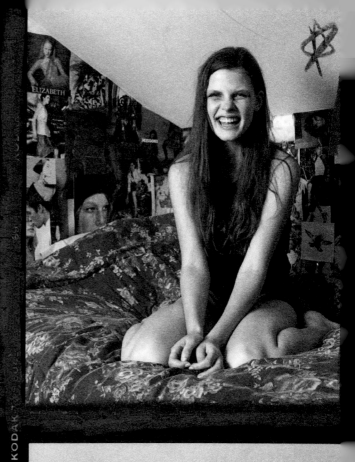
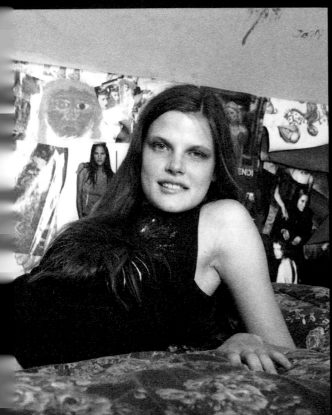
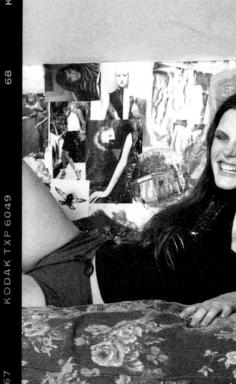

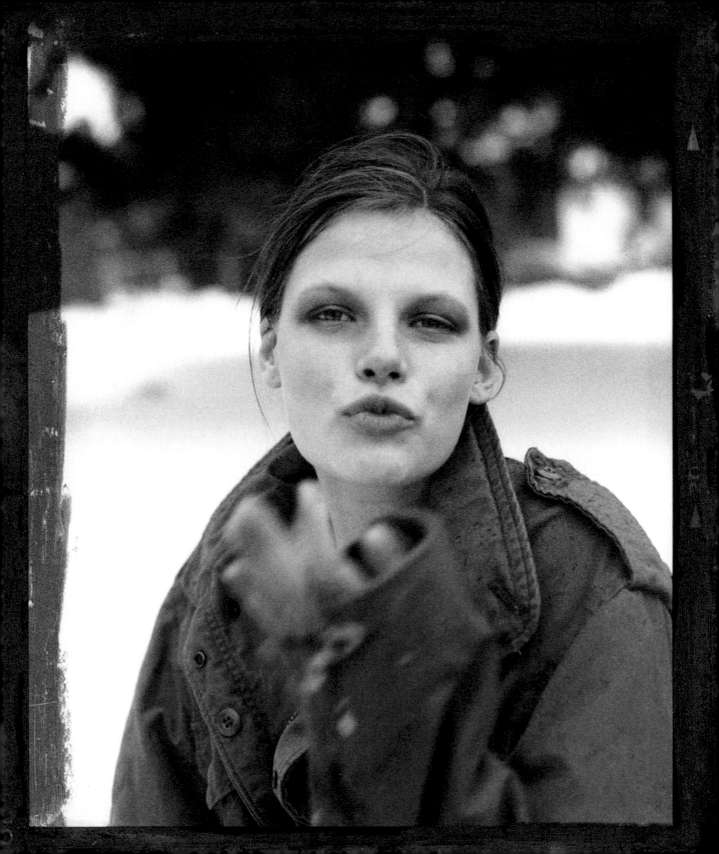

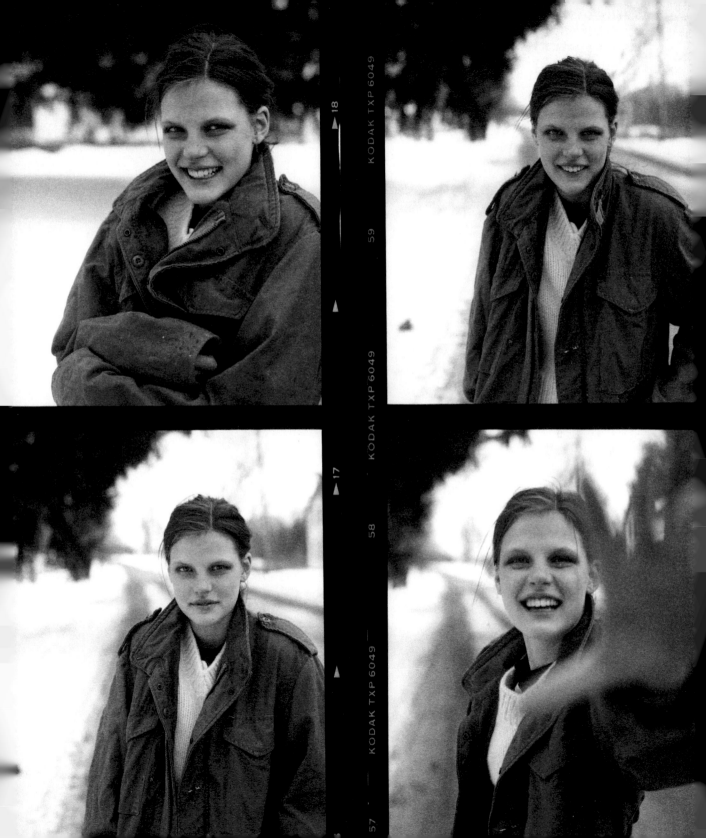

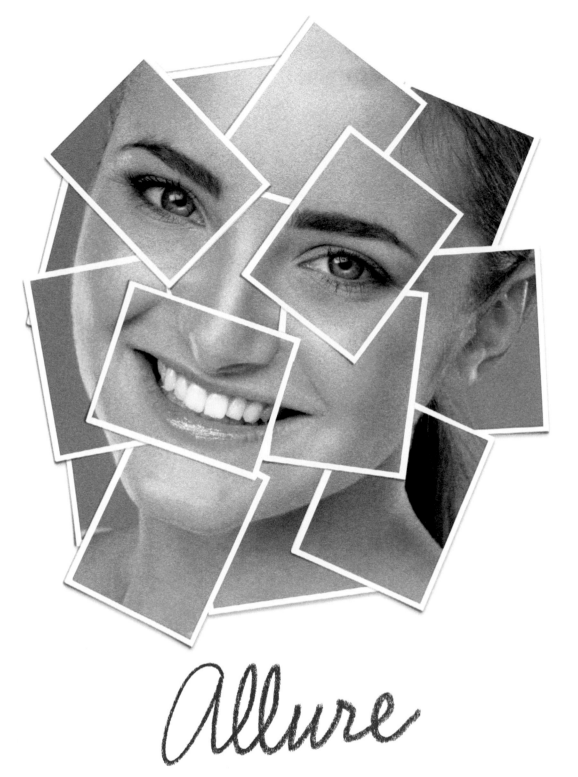

Allure

THE ABILITY TO ENTICE, INVITE, AND ATTRACT OTHERS

> "Beauty is a greater recommendation than any letter of introduction." —**Aristotle**

Casting Call: *the teach*

YOU'VE GOT THE PART!

Life. You've only got one. And guess what? You've got the part! You were born to play it. The greatest single casting call of your existence has been made, and you are the star. Are you going to accept the role of a lifetime and play the part to your fullest ability? Of course you are! You don't want to end up on the cutting-room floor—you want to walk the red carpet at the Academy Awards. You want to make the most of your life and live up to all of the potential that's inside you.

YO, I'LL TELL YOU WHAT I WANT, WHAT I REALLY, REALLY WANT

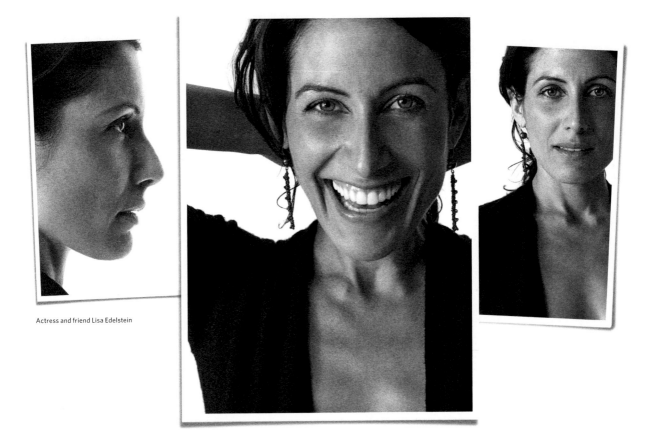

Actress and friend Lisa Edelstein

Every day, no matter where we go or who we see, we are being judged by the people around us on a "first impression" basis. Think about it. You do it too. When you pass a stranger on the street or meet someone new at a party, in class, or at a work function, your first impulse is to size that person up. What are they wearing? Is their hair styled or messy? Do they smile easily or purse their lips unintentionally? Do they seem approachable or do they make you want to turn and run?

In my business, models go on dozens of go-sees, auditions, and castings a day. Landing a modeling job is no easy feat. There are thousands of aspiring models and the competition is staggering. It may take hundreds of attempts for a girl to land an actual booking and a paycheck. So what makes one person get chosen over all the countless other wannabes who get sent home, licking their wounds?

More importantly, in your life challenges, how do you walk away as the chosen one instead of the wannabe?

> "I don't like that man. I must get to know him better." —Abraham Lincoln

Imagine walking into a room and there they are: the judges. There's the nice one (to give you encouragement), the experienced one (to offer up sage advice), and the mean one (to dish out the honest truth, no holds barred). Suddenly, like a bad dream, they all morph into versions of you, looking back at yourself.

That's right. I'm going to ask you to look at yourself as others might judge you upon first meeting you. And I'm going to challenge you to see both the places where you could use improvement and your undeniable strengths. Without being either too negative or too self-congratulatory, I want you to paint a clear picture of how others see you. Do you want to better yourself and be the most beautiful you? Then it's time to turn the judges' eyes on yourself. That doesn't mean you need to be critical. It means you need to be honest.

Again, we can learn from what models go through when they go on those hundreds of casting calls, because no matter how pretty they are, they don't always get the job. In fact, there is a lot of rejection. For some, the rejection proves to be too much. The girl who takes the words *no* and *pass* to heart isn't fit for fashion. But the girl who doesn't take rejection personally comes to grasp very quickly how to size up a room and learn from her mistakes. When she makes it to the top, it's because she knows herself well enough to become an expert at putting her best foot forward at all times.

You want to be *that* girl.

Why? Because over the years, how many times will you have to "audition"? Put another way, how many parties will you have to walk into where you have to overcome your insecurities? How many job interviews will you have to sweat through? How many times will you have to go on a first date?

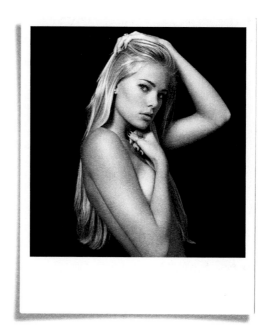

PROFILE IN ALLURE

TORI PRAVER

Tori Praver, the now-famous supermodel who has graced the cover of *Vogue* with her own exclusive line of swimwear, once upon a time sent a photo of herself to my studio saying she'd like to meet with me. Although she was represented by a small agency in Hawaii, she had no representation on the mainland. Now, I don't do this very often, but once in a while we do open calls to see new girls. Tori looked like she was worth meeting. When she arrived at the studio, we knew someone quite special had walked in. Not just because she was tall and modelesque, but because she had presence. At the tender age of eighteen, she was already charming; she could look you straight in the eye and, without any awkwardness, answer your questions; and after growing up on the beaches of Hawaii, she was quite happy in a swimsuit. Every test shot (like this one, from that very day) was a keeper and Tori was snapped up by the renowned modeling agency IMG immediately. And for this young starlet, the rest is history.

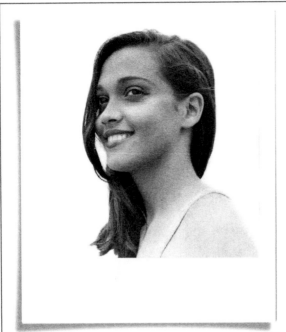
Gillian Barker, my mother

HISTORY'S MOST ALLURING WOMEN?

OUR MOTHERS!

My mom has always been one of those women who could walk into a room of strangers and command attention by doing little more than smiling. But she spent a lifetime doing much more than that. In the early 1960s, she won the Miss Sri Lanka title, only to have it stripped away because she wasn't 100 percent Sri Lankan. But that didn't stop her. She started modeling and, with her success, she moved herself, her sister, and my grandmother to England to start a new life. After working nonstop for decades in the entertainment and fashion industries as a singer and model, she went on to star in the most important role of her life, as a mother to four children—all while holding down a second job as the principal of a nursery school. She is a constant figure in my life, always encouraging me to dream. Her work ethic, combined with her ability to always be a lady, even in the toughest of scenarios, has taught and continues to teach me the meaning of allure. What do you find alluring about your mother?

LURING THEM WITH ALLURE

Do you remember the first time you met your best friend? How about your partner? What was it about your first impression of them that made you want to get to know them? It could be fascinating to evaluate whether or not they ultimately matched your first impression or whether they totally surprised you with something you didn't at first perceive. Regardless, though, at the time of that meeting, would you have ever gotten to know them better if they didn't have that initial allure?

In my line of work and during my travels, I meet wildly different people from all walks of life and all over the world, every day. And I'll be the first to attest, the old adage "You can't judge a book by its cover" is without a doubt true. But the topic at hand is first impressions, and a book's cover can definitely influence your decision as to whether you're going to read that book or another one. Sometimes people miss a book they would have really enjoyed just because it didn't make a good first impression.

You don't want to be *that* book.

What we are talking about here is allure. The ability to entice, invite, and attract others to want to know you.

THERE ARE NO RULES

I have a good friend (who shall remain nameless, to protect the innocent). By most accounts, when it comes to outward appearances, he most decidedly does *not* make a good first impression. He's a rather large, unkempt man who spends very little time on his personal hygiene, stuffs his face with hot dogs, and is basically an oafish slob. But once he opens his mouth to talk, a sparkle shines through his eyes. And he can tell a story better than anyone I've ever met. Within moments of his being at a party, a crowd gathers around him and people are hoping he'll choose them to be his friend. Now that's allure.

In other words, first impressions are not just about looks. They are about your charisma, your inner glow, your ability to draw people to you. I recently did a

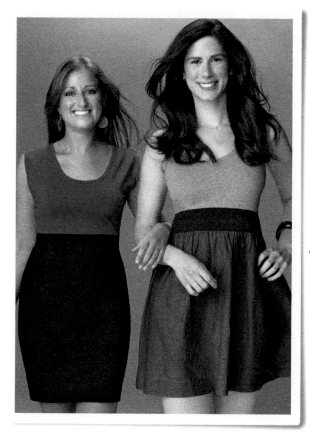

"Inner beauty and confidence start by surrounding yourself with positive people who encourage you to be yourself."

—Alexis Farah, associate beauty editor, *Women's Health* (right), with best friend, Marla Goldsmith

casting call where a young woman walked through the door who everyone thought was physically wrong for the job. As the casting progressed, I discovered something in her that I wanted to see more of. The test shoot began and we had an instant rapport. Because of this, her pictures were fabulously engaging. She booked the job on my insistence and, in the end, wowed the clients with her ability to deliver exactly what they wanted.

When I'm looking to cast a model for a campaign, I'm looking for a fantastic first impression, no matter what it might be. Maybe it's her charming wit, her simple sense of style, or her self-knowing charisma. Maybe it's some poetry I happen to catch her reading, or even her fabulously chosen scarf. The world of fashion moves at the speed of light, as does most of the working world in today's plugged-in, high-tech universe; while it would be wonderful to be able to sit down, have a nice chat, and really get to know each and every prospect,

that's not going to happen. And since you may not get that chance either when it comes to your own life's "auditions," the first impression you make counts.

That said, when casting I like to think that I don't necessarily know what I'm looking for. Although first impressions are important, they are often misleading. I try to look past the facade. Many aspiring models have no idea how to dress, walk, speak, or present themselves. On *America's Next Top Model* (*ANTM*), it has been my job to find the diamond in the rough, and through constructive criticism and a series of teaches and challenges, help them show us whether or not they have modeling potential.

Think of yourself as being at that point. You're not supposed to be a working model already. In fact, you may have no modeling aspirations whatsoever. You're trying to discover and reveal your allure. What is it about you and within you that is enticing, inviting, and attractive?

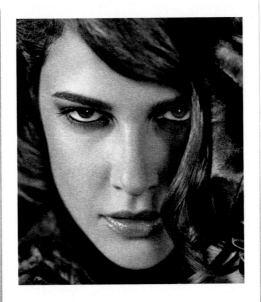

THE GIRL
CAN'T HELP IT

KATARINA SCOLA

Sometimes someone turns up for an audition and, despite the fact that they aren't what you are looking for, they lure you in. Katarina Scola walked into our casting and, although she was a little older and more exotic than the creative brief we were working with called for, she blew us away. She oozed confidence and could stare my camera down as if her life depended on it. Although we had seen more than a hundred girls for the shoot, it was clear Katarina was the one.

THERE ARE *SOME* RULES

"Do I contradict myself?
Very well then I contradict myself, (I am large, I contain multitudes.)" —*Song of Myself*, Walt Whitman

Perhaps the first thing that catches my eye when a girl walks in for a casting is her outfit. Does she look put-together and elegant, or does she look like she just finished her spinning class and has rushed over from the gym? So, when it comes to making a good first impression, on the one hand, there are no rules (because human beings are fascinating on many levels), but on the other, some rules are universal truths.

YOU ARE WHAT YOU WEAR

Wear clothes that correspond to the occasion. If you are going to a job interview at a company, dress like you already work there. If you are going to a formal dinner at the Four Seasons, don't wear jeans and a T-shirt. And if you are going to the mall, wear jeans and a T-shirt, not a tube top and short shorts. It boils down to good old-fashioned common sense. It's important to wear what you like and feel good in, but it's equally important to make a first impression that communicates that you want to be where you are.

YOU CAN NEVER GO WRONG WITH BASICS

The simple black dress works well for many women. Basics are solid and simple and can be formal or casual. Learn to know what you look good in. What colors complement your skin tone? What colors make your eyes pop? It's always a good idea to wear clothes that fit and flatter your body type. Clothes that are too tight or too baggy are distracting. Clothes that are too trendy are generally unimpressive as well, because the look has already been done before by too many.

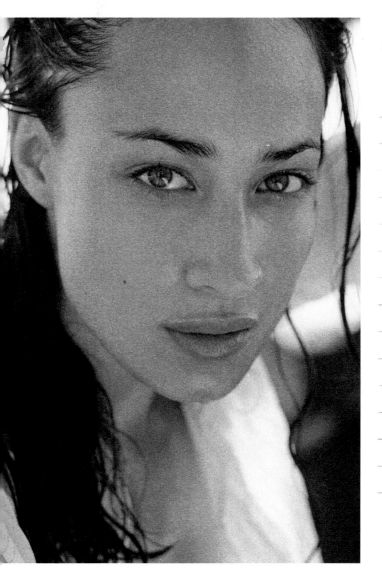

Quick List
Making a Good Impression

These things may seem obvious, but you'd be amazed at how many people forget them under pressure.

1. Be neat, clean, and groomed
2. Stand up straight
3. Make eye contact
4. Listen
5. Smile!

"Allure to me is sharing something personal about myself without speaking a word, being vulnerable and courageous at the same time. Allure is subtle, beautiful, sweet, and mysterious."

—Crissy Barker, my wife

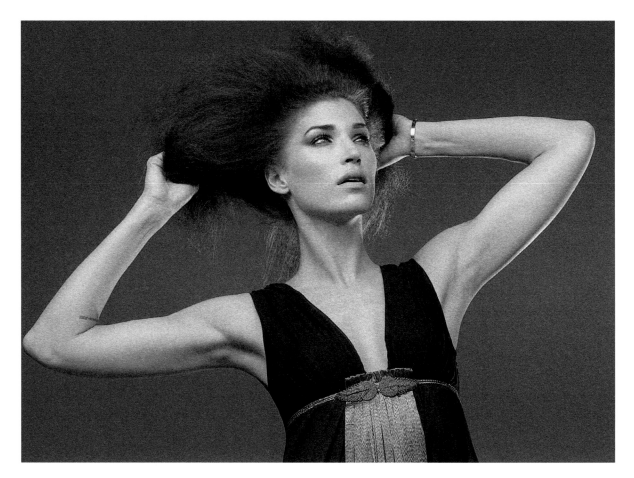

"Your hair reflects who you are, but you should own your natural hair and embrace it. Great hair can make you feel like an entirely different person. Whenever I get my hair blown out, I call it 'sex hair.' It makes me feel beautiful and sexy!" —*ANTM* contestant Ann Markley

LESS IS MORE

When it looks like you've been at home adding more accessories, more makeup, and more hair spray, it looks like you are trying too hard, and just not nailing it. Sometimes too much effort shows—and the effect is not always a winner. How do you know when enough is enough? Best to be ruled by instinct and intuition, though I have a friend who says you should take one accessory *off* before you walk out the door.

WANNA BE ON TOP? BE A HAIR ABOVE THE REST

Hair is part of your ensemble. What's the point of having a smashing outfit and then having your hair look a mess? Here too, simple is superior. Your hair is the frame of your face, and your face is your masterpiece. Rarely does a fine work of art look better in an ornate, over-the-top frame; that just competes with the painting. Same goes for your features. Too much height and poof in your hair sidetracks us from the main attraction: *you*. When in doubt, put your hair in a bun. It's a foolproof remedy for bad hair days and gives you an instantly chic hairstyle.

LEAVE YOUR BAGGAGE AT HOME

Having a bad day? We all have them. We face the morning and, whether we've been up all night or not, we just don't feel 100 percent. Maybe there was a phone call from someone we didn't want to hear from, or maybe we're sick, or we've lost something special. It *matters* how you feel. Always evaluate what is important to you. But when you are going anywhere for a possible opportunity, never go filled with excuses. People care, but not when there's a job or other opportunity at stake. How many times do we watch reality television and someone says they are not at their best because of blah, blah, blah. "I'm sick." "My boyfriend broke up with me on Twitter." You *know* what we all think when we are watching those shows: "Poor girl, she's about to be sent home!"

All things taken seriously, take all things seriously. If things are really that bad, stay at home. Don't show up and make others feel sorry for you. However, if you are sick, take care of yourself! We all know our limits. If you are "sick" (i.e., just feeling "off" but not actually, physically ill), time to push forward and do your best. There is no shame in canceling an engagement because you really can't make it. There is shame in showing up and then saying, "I'm perfect for this opportunity, but you caught me at a bad time." That's not the way things work in any field. No employer will ever be impressed if you show up a wreck, saying you aren't at your best because your cat is dying. They'll wonder why you aren't at home with your cat.

EVEN FANS SHOULDN'T FAWN

You are out to impress; you're not desperate. I'm naturally attracted to shooting someone who comes in and is eager to work. Employers want to hire someone who wants the job. But when someone is too eager to laugh at my jokes and too quick to pay me a compliment, I become wary.

If you are honestly impressed with someone, praise is not out of the question, but being a fan is about showing respect. You are qualified. You are perfect for the job and the embodiment of what they are looking for. Own it. But don't overdo it.

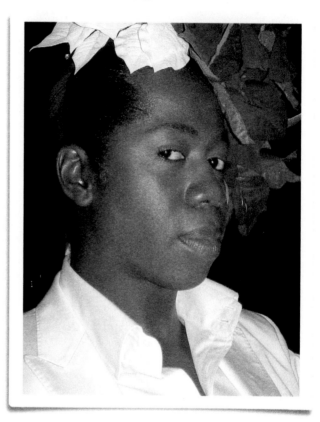

"Girl, once you kiss someone's ass to get something, if you get it, break out the ChapStick, because you're going to have to keep kissing that ass until a better ass-kisser comes along. Snap!"
—*ANTM* judge Miss J. Alexander

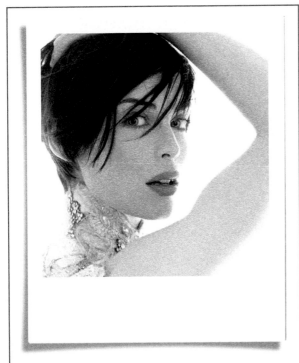

ALLURE IN THE HOUSE

YOANNA HOUSE

"Allure is mystery. It's not giving it all away. No matter what age you are, I think it's always great to leave a sense of mystery so people will always want more. Especially men. They love that."

If you are going to go on national television to compete in a modeling competition, go prepared! Yoanna House was, and I was especially impressed with her. To this day she eats, sleeps, and breathes fashion. She has the names of all the leading models on the tip of her tongue, always knows a photographer's work, and is familiar with most well-known designers. She makes a fantastic first impression, always. She is a winner, due largely to her ease with and knowledge of the world she is pursuing. Just being good-looking never qualifies you for a job. You have to work. But if you love your work, it's easy.

KNOW YOUR STUFF

All too often, we turn up for important opportunities ill-prepared. When going in for a job interview, don't you want to know enough about the company or institution to be able to talk comfortably about how you can contribute? When you are meeting your partner's family, wouldn't you rather bring flowers they love than take a stab in the dark and perhaps even offend someone? It's your one shot. Make it count. Take the time to be prepared. Sheer fabulousness alone no longer cuts it!

I can't tell you how often I advise hopeful models to study magazines and books on fashion and photography. Girls still come in, some a little cocky, unable to tell you who Kate Moss or Isaac Mizrahi is—and those are some heavy hitters in the fashion world. In fact, I'd venture to say they are household names; at a casting call, I'd expect you to have heard of them and have a basic awareness of who they are, even if all you have been doing is glancing at tabloids on the supermarket checkout line or shopping at Target! The point is, how could you ever expect to apply for and land a job in a field you don't know even the most rudimentary things about? Bottom line: The more prepared you are, the better you'll feel about yourself in any new situation.

FAILURE IS NOT AN OPTION

Don't give yourself any reason to fail. When you are going anywhere, especially someplace where making a great first impression counts, make sure you are prepared not just mentally but also physically and tactically. Get off to a good start; make sure you've had a meal that will sustain you and give you energy. You want time on your side, so don't linger in front of the mirror too long or fool about on Facebook until you're running late. Make sure you've got everything you might need by going through a "just in case" checklist. Keep your composure by knowing you have your favorite makeup items, a mirror for touch-ups, and tissues for a sudden sneeze. Rely on yourself for that bottle of water for a dry throat instead of hoping one will be offered to you. The more obstacles you eliminate for yourself, the more composed you will be, and the more you will hold the reins and keep your eyes on the prize.

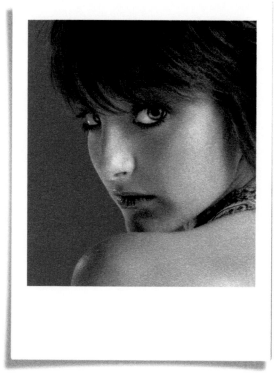

Photographed five years ago for the Make-A-Wish Foundation

THROUGH HER EYES

NICOLE RAY MULLER

"At the age of 13, I was diagnosed with cancer and stripped of everything I had physically. I had to focus on what was inside. I was forced to face the girl within me."

I first met Nicole Ray Muller when photographing her for the Make-A-Wish Foundation. Then, at age 14, she was bravely undergoing surgeries and chemotherapy treatments in an effort to save her life. Amidst the uncertainty of her disease, Nicole's wish was to be a supermodel for a day; and I was more than happy to fulfill it. When she arrived on set, I was immediately drawn to her. Although frail from the treatments, she had a driving presence that shone through her eyes, and she quickly captivated the entire studio. Her gaze revealed her journey and, although filled with pain, it was also full of strength and determination.

I was thrilled to be able to invite Nicole back, five years later, to be photographed for the *Beauty Equation*. Now in remission, the difference in her physical appearance is striking—her face is fuller, her smile unconcerned, and her health abundant. A 19-year-old college student, Nicole is full of life. I selected her photograph as the opening image of this chapter because her eyes not only tell the story of a survivor but also because her natural allure remains present in both hardship and recovery. The epitome of a girl who speaks volumes with her eyes, Nicole makes you want to get to know her, and lucky for us, it looks like there will be many, many years for us to do just that.

GET OUT OF YOUR OWN WAY

Courage is not the absence of fear; it is the conquest of it. In the fashion industry, models line up at a casting to have their every angle scrutinized by the client. They have five minutes to leave a lasting impression that will book a job. Picture yourself in that position.

Nervous yet?

Everybody is. And there is no remedy but confidence—which we'll get to shortly. Everyone has nerves. We're all human, after all. Sometimes nerves get the best of us and we don't make the impression we want to make. Don't let your nervousness hold you back. How many times have you relived a moment in your head and then wished you had the chance to go back with the confidence you gained in hindsight? You know now exactly what you would have said, recognize what you could have avoided revealing, or realize what you should have worn. Would have, could have, should have. Relax. Keep in mind that everyone's in the same boat. The goal is to present your best self, especially on a first impression. Whatever happens, don't project a negative self-image. Everyone screws up now and then. Learn from experience and do better next time. Always give yourself a break. It's really never the end of the world, no matter how many times you experience rejection. And there's no foul for not hitting a home run your first time at bat.

It is always puzzling when we have girls who come to the show, especially the elimination, looking like they are in a streetwalking competition instead of a modeling competition! Even in a professional casting session, I might give a mini-makeover right there in the room, usually by removing an item or twelve. Girls come in with a tonnage of accessories and hair that resembles a fright wig on a drag queen, looking like they are ready for a big night eating chips and watching wrestling on TV, or committing any number of fashion infractions that are all remedied with a little common sense. And then there's my pet peeve, which goes by the term we have coined as *hoochie*.

In the 1960s and '70s, the women's movement spearheaded a campaign to liberate women—a fight that has gone on for centuries. Remember that women couldn't vote in the United States until Susan B. Anthony and the suffragists ultimately changed all that by getting the Nineteenth Amendment to the Constitution passed in 1920. Just thirty years ago, women were still fighting to end the constant and insidious objectification of women as sex objects for men. Although a lot has changed since then, it sometimes seems like much of that pioneering work gets thrown out the window by the granddaughters of the women who fought for a woman's right to own her sexuality.

Be sexual and be sexy! It's sensational. It's sexational! But the trend of being *hoochie* needs to stop. The media has embraced Madonna, Britney Spears, and Lady Gaga for their provocative and in-your-face sexual bravado. That's pop music and tabloid glitz. In real life, it's simply not acceptable to be in public dressed like a two-bit hooker. It's inappropriate and just plain trashy. Dressing modestly doesn't mean dressing like a nun. But exposing too much skin in public is often unattractive, out of place, and uncomfortable for others. If you have a great figure or a flat stomach, fantastic—go to the beach, where a bikini is the appropriate attire. It's all about context. Exposed midriffs may be currently in fashion, but for interviews and auditions, the workplace, or even the department store, please make sure your top reaches your bottom. And there are extremely few circumstances where it is appropriate to wear low-cut jeans that expose your lacy thong. Sexy is a state of mind, not a state of undress.

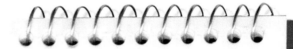

Quick List
Avoiding the H-Word Label

Here are some common-sense tips to ensure your integrity doesn't end up in the good taste lost-and-found.

1. Visible bras and thongs belong in the bedroom, not the boardroom
2. Too short, too tight, or too low cut: It's all too much
3. Beware the VPL (visible panty line)
4. Keep your private piercings private
5. An exposed midsection expands your hoochie quotient

A FINAL WORD— DON'T MISCAST YOURSELF!

Casting is all about finding the right person to represent a role. We've all been to a film where we thought, "She's not right for that part!" That's called miscasting. It happens all the time. There are some rare actors

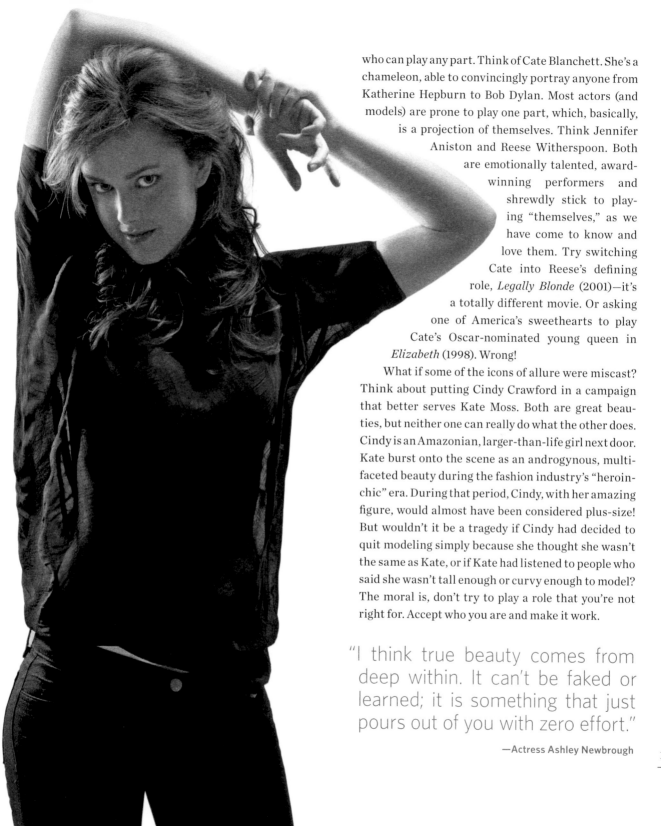

who can play any part. Think of Cate Blanchett. She's a chameleon, able to convincingly portray anyone from Katherine Hepburn to Bob Dylan. Most actors (and models) are prone to play one part, which, basically, is a projection of themselves. Think Jennifer Aniston and Reese Witherspoon. Both are emotionally talented, award-winning performers and shrewdly stick to playing "themselves," as we have come to know and love them. Try switching Cate into Reese's defining role, *Legally Blonde* (2001)—it's a totally different movie. Or asking one of America's sweethearts to play Cate's Oscar-nominated young queen in *Elizabeth* (1998). Wrong!

What if some of the icons of allure were miscast? Think about putting Cindy Crawford in a campaign that better serves Kate Moss. Both are great beauties, but neither one can really do what the other does. Cindy is an Amazonian, larger-than-life girl next door. Kate burst onto the scene as an androgynous, multi-faceted beauty during the fashion industry's "heroin-chic" era. During that period, Cindy, with her amazing figure, would almost have been considered plus-size! But wouldn't it be a tragedy if Cindy had decided to quit modeling simply because she thought she wasn't the same as Kate, or if Kate had listened to people who said she wasn't tall enough or curvy enough to model? The moral is, don't try to play a role that you're not right for. Accept who you are and make it work.

"I think true beauty comes from deep within. It can't be faked or learned; it is something that just pours out of you with zero effort."

—Actress Ashley Newbrough

Now for the fun stuff! Pull out those initial self-portraits you took. This is going to be page one of your workbook—whether it be an actual notebook or your post on www.beautyequation.com. Put your self-portraits there, at the beginning, with nothing else. And with that, your journey has begun.

1. TAKE THE OATH!

"Honesty is an active verb, not a passive noun. Go out of your way to be truthful, beginning with the things that you say to yourself."

— Joe Tye, America's Values Coach

I want you to tell the truth, the whole truth, and nothing but the truth. The challenge here is to be honest with yourself. And by asking you to be honest, I am not asking you to be harsh and overly critical. I want you to think frankly about yourself, without attacking. You are just having a conversation with yourself, not your friends, your parents, or your partner. You are your own best friend. You can confide in yourself. You can compliment yourself. You can critique yourself. But above all, be truthful with yourself.

1. This first bit should be easy, because most of us are very hard on ourselves. You're the "mean judge." Write down five things about yourself that you could easily improve with a little effort. They can be about your physical appearance or your personality. Write!

2. This part might be a little harder, because most of us have trouble complimenting and encouraging ourselves. You're the "nice judge." Write down five things that you feel are your most important physical attributes. What makes you unique and helps you make a good first impression? Is it your great, untamed hair; your crooked but winning smile; your youthful dimples? Write!

3. Now, the hardest part of all, because it requires tapping into the kind of perspective we usually use on others, not ourselves. You're the "experienced judge." Offer yourself what you would consider sage advice. Write down five things that you feel are your most important emotional attributes, whether or not they need some improvement. What are the things inside that you feel rub people the right way when you meet them? Are you a great conversationalist, a good listener, or exceedingly funny? Write!

Well done—you've just described your allure! Some of it may need a bit of a boost, but that's why you're doing the Beauty Equation.

2. UNFORGETTABLE

You are about to take another self-portrait. But first, take a moment and think about your most memorable quality. Feel free to think of several at first, and go ahead and write them all down where you are going to put this next photo; but in the end, you are going to pick just one quality to embody for this challenge. Try to remember if anyone has ever told you, "Oh yeah, I remember you. You had that infectious laugh" or "You looked amazing in that dress at the party last week. You have such good taste." Narrow it down to the one memorable thing about you that you are most comfortable with, remembering the secrets of your own allure from the previous writing challenge. Take a self-portrait!

3. WHAT'S YOUR HOOK?

What is the message you most want to portray about yourself? What is it that you want the world to know about you? What do you stand for? Do you want to change the world? How? Do you want to shout out to the world that you are a kind and caring person? Are you mad as hell and not going to take it anymore? Think about it, and let your heart do the talking. Take a self-portrait!

Time to get your camera out again. Fashion experts will agree that our eyes are the most important part of our overall package. That's why we all try to get models to "smile" with their eyes. You can say words with your eyes. Conversely, you can say absolutely nothing with them. One of the biggest problems some gorgeous models have is that when they get in front of a camera, their eyes become dead—usually because they don't have a thought in their pretty heads! I want you to think about one thing you want me to know about you. It could be anything: a crush, a dream, or the fact that you've just mastered making chocolate soufflé. Your challenge: Convey this to me through your eyes alone. Take a self-portrait!

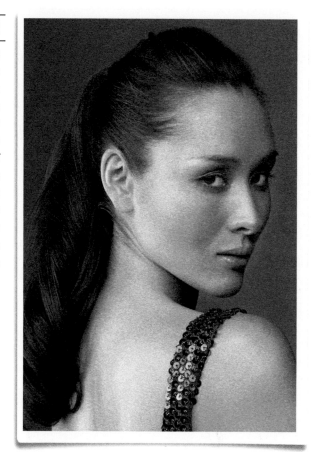

April Wilkner

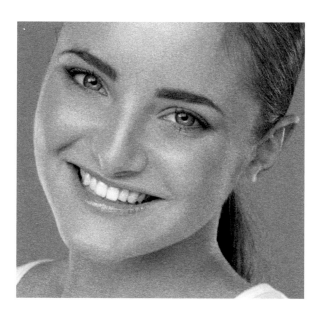

Nicole Ray Muller, nineteen, student, capturing allure

TODAY'S notion of beauty encompasses every size, shape, and color. The power of any given woman's personal allure is unstoppable. Go wrong and you can suffer the consequences of exaggeration, arrogance, and sluttishness. Go right and you can possess the formula for sincerity, integrity, and charm.

It's up to you to understand your own allure. It's your life and your starring role.

33

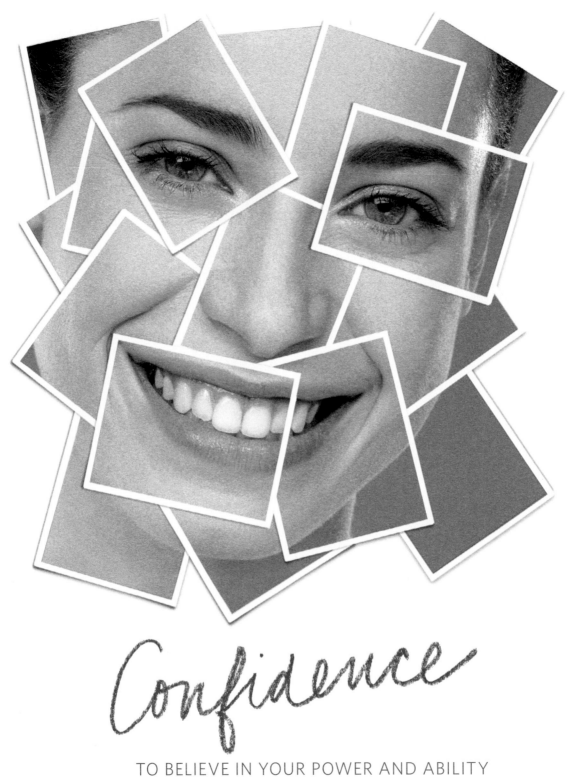

Confidence

TO BELIEVE IN YOUR POWER AND ABILITY

Lights, Camera, Action: *the teach*

YOU'RE ON!

"Action!" Its meaning is the same whether the context is the "tell us about yourself" at the start of a job interview, the "and just how did you meet our son?" on first sitting down with the boyfriend's folks, or the literal "lights, camera, action!" if you're lucky enough to be cast in a movie or TV show. Everything has built up to this moment and all eyes are on *you*!

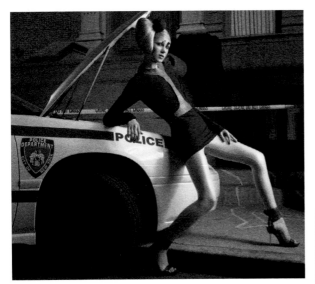

Rebecca Epley

It's easy to look, feel, and act confident when you know you're good at something. That's second nature. You stand up tall. You smile and laugh, even when things get difficult. You know what you want and have no problem asking for it. You aren't afraid to engage in conversation about what you're doing, because you know all about it. You feel no need to brag or self-aggrandize. You're "on." You can feel people responding to you. Makes you feel kind of sexy, doesn't it? Beautiful, even? Don't back down from that. You're allowed to feel good about being good at things.

But what about the vast amounts of things you fear you're not good at?

Your heart begins to pound. Drops of sweat materialize on your forehead. Suddenly you have an itch, perhaps a breakout of hives. You keep your arms clenched closely to your sides for fear your antiperspirant won't prevent unsightly spotting. Everything starts to get blurry, your vision narrows to black, and *kerplunk!* You keel over.

Over the years, I've seen all of this happen when judging the runway. One memorable girl, the gorgeous and usually vivacious Rebecca Epley, was having her photo evaluated, when suddenly her eyes rolled back and she fainted right there in front of the judges' panel and all the stunned girls. Ouch! No doubt, nerves played a part.

There's a lot of pressure on you when you take center stage. The pressure can lead to the nervous blunders that can deter you from the accomplishment that should be yours. But it doesn't need to be that way.

Believe it or not, you can learn how to transform the natural human condition of apprehension about new and different things into a positive. And once you master that, I promise that you'll feel your Beauty Equation climbing higher than ever.

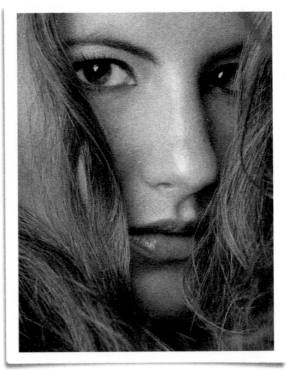

"Beauty is happiness. It's going a full day without receiving a single compliment and being 100 percent confident you look amazing."
—Heather Muir, beauty editor, *Seventeen* magazine

HARNESSING FEAR TO WRANGLE SUCCESS

We all know the quote from Franklin D. Roosevelt: "There is nothing to fear but fear itself." Why has this saying stood the test of time? Quite simply, because most things we fear are not as frightening as they seem. Problems start when you let what you are afraid of rule your behavior. Fear breeds insecurity; confidence comes from knowing you can overcome it. You want to exude confidence? Practice overcoming your fears!

When you embrace your fears by accepting and admitting that you are afraid of something (as opposed to running away or ignoring the fact), give yourself a well-deserved "congrats." Because you've won the first battle! The fear is no longer as large once the mystery has been dispelled.

Another great quote from the iconic American author Mark Twain: "Courage is not the absence of fear, but the mastery of fear." In other words, even the most courageous among us experience fear or nervousness. The trick is to master it, instead of letting it master you.

Don't forget that fear is also afraid of itself. Greet it by name and imagine yourself saying, "Hey, you! I see you there, and you can't scare me. I know you want me to run screaming from you, but I'm not going to. If you want a piece of me, bring it!" Fear can't stand up to that kind of awareness. Keep practicing this and, eventually, you'll transform your anxiety into an ability to rise to the occasion.

This is my challenge to you. Embrace your fears as an avenue to self-confidence. If you can channel them, you will turn your nerves into a raw energy that will give you the strength to step into the outside world with a vibrant, heightened sensitivity.

HISTORY'S MOST CONFIDENT WOMAN?

HELEN KELLER

"Security is mostly a superstition. It does not exist in nature, nor do the children of men as a whole experience it. Avoiding danger is no safer in the long run than outright exposure. Life is either a daring adventure, or nothing."

Despite being deaf and blind, Helen Keller was a prolific American author, lecturer, and political activist. She was the first person who was deaf and blind to earn a Bachelor of Arts degree.

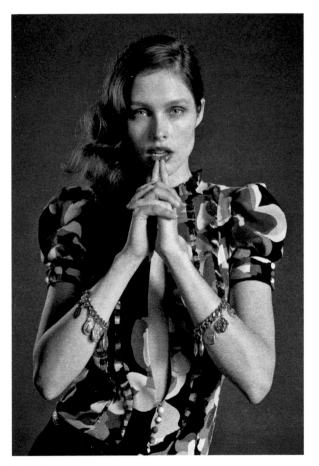

Lonneke Engel

"There is a misconception that women would not be able to handle a 3,500–pound race car with 850+ horsepower. Exuding confidence and strength in everything: posture, walking, talking, handling critics, handling fans. . . that has been a huge plus."

—Jennifer Jo Cobb, NASCAR racer

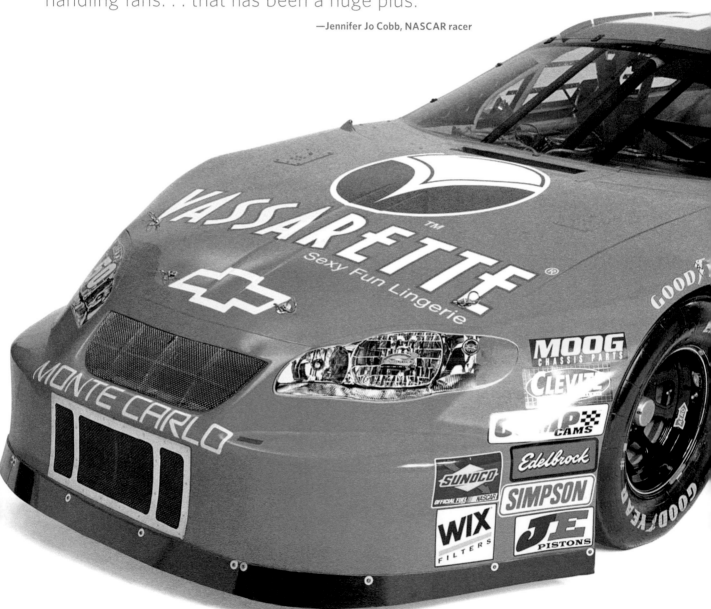

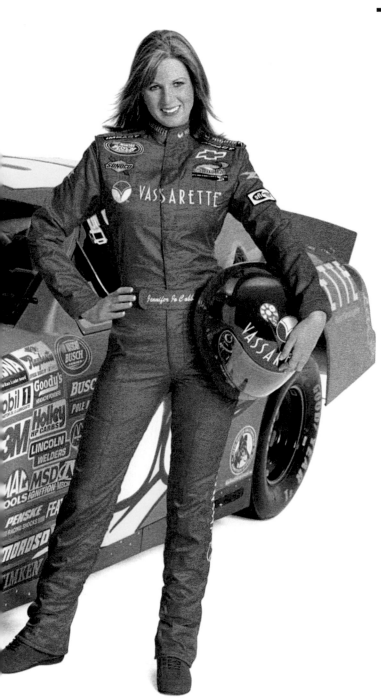

STEPPING ON THE GAS,
OR PEDAL TO THE METAL

I consider myself a confident person. It's something I've worked on and developed over many years of self-reflection. It takes experience and drive to succeed in my business. That's not to say I don't still get a little nervous when I am in the spotlight and I hear the words "Action! All eyes on you, Nigel!" Gulp.

It's like being behind the wheel at the start of a race. The red light is holding you back; it's about to turn green. You get butterflies in your stomach wondering what you're going to do when the light changes. Will you have the guts to gun it and roar away to victory, seeing the checkered flag wave for you at the finish line? Or will you creep forward and let everyone pass you by? Life waits for no one. If you are not going to have the confidence to look straight ahead and say, "I know where I'm going!" well, then you might as well just close your eyes, scream, and drift out into the oncoming traffic, hoping for the best.

Personally, through channeling my nerves and having faith in my own ability to succeed, even when I have never tried something before, I usually find the confidence I need. A few years back, I made my "acting" debut on the soap opera *The Young and the Restless*. Granted, I was playing a role I'm usually very good at: a noted fashion photographer named Nigel Barker. I arrived on set and must admit that my adrenaline was rushing. I had to stay focused on not letting my nerves get the best of me. I've spent hours in front of the camera as a model and, of course as a judge on *ANTM*. But this was a little different—now I was working with a director, other actors, and a script. I took a deep breath and I told myself that I had already memorized my lines. I had come prepared. I'd been visualizing what the experience would be like in my head and, so far, the day had met all my expectations. No jarring surprises or curveballs. I relaxed and did the job I knew I could do. It ended up being a delightful experience and it was an invaluable deposit into my realm of knowledge.

BASIC EQUIPMENT IN THE WAR AGAINST NERVES

KNOW YOUR MACHINE

Do you know what actually happens when we get nervous? The body releases adrenaline, which is produced by the aptly named adrenal gland, and this physically affects the body—increased heart rate, blushing, problems breathing, perspiration, butterflies, and any number of physical quirks and ticks appear out of nowhere. Adrenaline is naturally produced in high-stress or physically exhilarating situations. It's your body's way of assisting you when you need that little extra lift to do something special, like meet a new group of people, ace an interview, or speak before a large audience.

Yet many of us find adrenaline to be the "enemy" that keeps us down, because we don't understand what happens to us when we become nervous. Adrenaline is like a gift from your body that boosts your normal functions. Think about the adrenaline rush you get after a roller coaster ride or a first kiss with someone you've got a massive crush on. The trouble is, the body sends adrenaline out in heightened situations *both positive and negative.*

If you can anticipate the effects adrenaline will have on you, you won't feel so helpless when it appears in moments when you feel stressed. This is not a standardized measure in humans; everyone is different and every adrenal gland has its own routine that is specific to your body. Since you have been driving your own model of your human machine since you were born, only you know what to expect. You need to make note of how you personally react so that, when it happens, you have more control over it. Knowing what to expect has a huge impact on our comfort and confidence levels.

If drinking coffee or energy drinks tends to increase the negative effect adrenaline has on you, drink water! But if such beverages lift you up and give you the edge you need, stop for an espresso on your way. Does a cup of hot tea, cocoa, or milk soothe your nerves? Sounds like a good idea.

DON'T FORGET TO BREATHE!

Adrenaline rushes often constrict the windpipes, veins, and lungs, resulting in troubled breathing. Sometimes, when we get that rush, we may even forget to breathe entirely. Make sure you check to see if you are holding your breath by accident. In these moments, it is important to remind your body to do its duty and take in nice, long, slow, deep breaths.

Practice now: Take a long, deep breath and then try to exhale taking twice as long. This has proven effective in lowering your heart rate and creating a greater sense of calm.

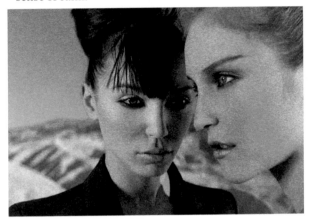

Stephanie Wood and Ruby Corley

REMEMBER, A JEDI IS ALWAYS PREPARED

Knowledge is power. Power is knowledge. As I have mentioned before, a few hours or even a few minutes of research will give you the edge you need to walk into any room with increased confidence. Educate yourself about who you are going to meet and what you are going to be discussing. That said, no one's ever going to expect you know everything; it's always better to admit you don't know something and ask a good question than to wing it and possibly come off looking silly. It quickly becomes very obvious when you are pretending to be something you are not or when you are exaggerating your skill sets. And, truthfully, there's no better way to make yourself implode with insecurity than to try to fake knowing something you know absolutely nothing about. Prepare. And be honest and open when you need help.

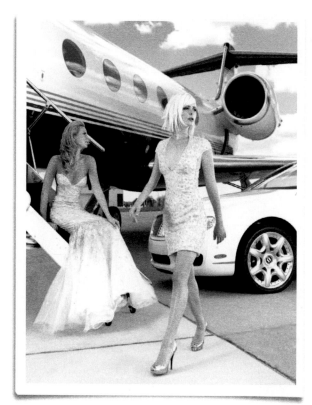

"True beauty is having faith in yourself and having the confidence to present yourself at your best." —Sydney DeVos, nineteen, aspiring actress and student (right), with her sister, Cassandra DeVos

Many doctors and health organizations trumpet that music has a great effect on the body, and we all know its effect on our souls. Some say that fast music increases metabolism and muscular energy, steps up the heartbeat, sends a rush of blood to the brain, and elevates blood pressure. Slow, peaceful music, they espouse, can produce calm, but can also make you feel still and inactive. Soft music has a definite anesthetic effect and there have even been claims that it dulls mild sensations of pain.

So can music help you improve your confidence? Pump up the jam. You bet it can! Some music can just make you feel good, and it tends to make you feel more comfortable with who you are. Music that soothes and relaxes you turns off all the negative voices of worry and doubt in your mind and helps to you maintain your composure. Again, only you know what works, because you march to the beat of your own drummer.

On a recent assignment, I was photographing a girl who was having a lackluster shoot. She was feeling, by her own account, insecure, dull, and listless. I asked her what was wrong and she said she couldn't wrap her head around it. I asked her if she had a favorite song she could think about. Luckily, she did. Not only did thinking about the song totally relax her, but it filled her eyes with content and we had a great shoot. It made me realize another simple thing you should always travel with: your own theme song!

Start taking note: Do you have a song that makes you happy every time you hear it? Is there a song you sing in your head that gives you courage or takes your mind off your fear? What would you sing before you're about to run a race? How about when you're on your way to confront a person you have an issue with? What kind of song might make you feel more confident?

Take some time to listen to your music collection and find a song that can be your "confidence theme song." Let this song empower you every time you listen to it on your portable music player. Take this song with you everywhere in your brain and use it whenever your confidence needs a boost!

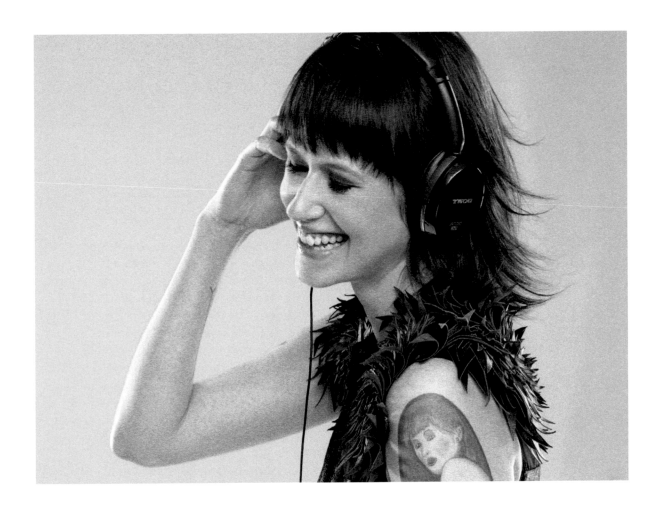

🎧

(DOWNLOAD)

SONGS ABOUT CONFIDENCE

"I'm every woman, it's all in me!"

"I'm Every Woman"— CHAKA KHAN

"Independent Women"— DESTINY'S CHILD

"Miss Independent"— KELLY CLARKSON

"I Will Survive"— GLORIA GAYNOR

"We Got the Beat"— THE GO-GO'S

"Music makes you feel empowered! There is nothing better than walking down the street and listening to eighties music. It can make you walk a little taller, stand a littler straighter, and put a little swing in your step."

—*ANTM* contestant Shandi Sullivan

BASIC EQUIPMENT
IN THE FIGHT TO GAIN CONFIDENCE

LATHER, RINSE, REPEAT

Let's forget about fear for a moment and think instead about being good at things, because that's when we really shine, right? So, first question: How does anyone get better at anything?

Answer: repetition.

That's why athletes are great role models on how to build confidence. When an athlete sets out to conquer a sport, like tennis or ice-skating, the first things they learn are what muscles they are going to rely on. U.S. Open and Wimbledon champ Maria Sharapova needs a powerful shoulder muscle to deliver a killer tennis serve, just like Guinness World Record holder and professional figure skater Lucinda Ruh needs intense thigh muscles to hold on to her trademark world's fastest and longest spin. Once they identify the muscles they will be relying on, athletes develop them, working them over and over again. Muscle learns strength through repetition, and the more athletes focus on these muscles through practice, the more they can be confident they will be able to do what they need them to do. As any pro athlete will tell you, there is a not much that separates people at the top. The difference between a journeyman/woman player and an elite player mirrors one of the key differences between a pretty girl and a beautiful woman: confidence.

Think of confidence as a muscle you need to develop so it will be strong, agile, and ready to use when you need it. Identify your insecurities. Do you have trouble making and keeping eye contact? Do you speak softly? Do you fidget or bite your nails when the pressure is on? Take those insecurities and practice conquering them; tell them what you want them to do. It's a fun workout and you don't even have to go to the gym! Work with someone you are comfortable with, a pal. Look them in the eye and engage in a conversation. If your eyes wander, start over. Practice being in control of your eye contact until you know you've mastered it. And then, reward yourself. Pat yourself on the back. From now

on, always remember when you go out in the world that eye contact is a piece of cake, because you've put in the work and have the confidence you need!

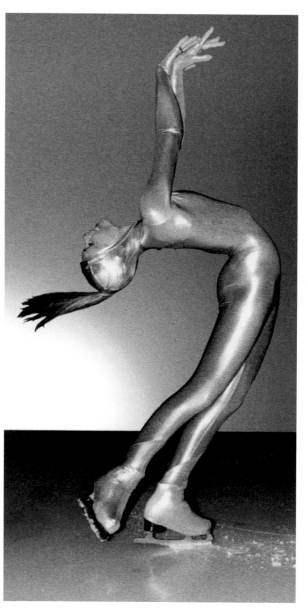

Lucinda Ruh, from a photo shoot for *Paper* magazine

When taking the portrait of an actor, dancer, athlete, or young model just starting their career, I often have to help them build up their confidence (further evidence that no matter what level of fame you've achieved in your field, when you step onto unfamiliar turf, the confidence that has served you so well elsewhere can take a beating).

In fact, actors often are not at ease being themselves in front of the camera. They're used to developing other characters and playing them for the lens. It's easier for them to "perform" than to "be." That's not to say a great shot can't be had when someone is playing a character. But a fictional character is not the essence of who someone really is, or the essence of a beautiful portrait.

Confidence is not acting. It's being. It's believing in yourself, not in a projection of what you think others want you to be.

BANKING ON CONFIDENCE

TYRA BANKS

Tyra is the portrait of self-confidence at its best. She's a paragon of the words *fearless, friendly,* and *fierce.* Think of her and you will have an inner role model of someone who exudes confidence in a way that adds to her beauty.

The first African-American woman to appear on the cover of the *Sports Illustrated* swimsuit issue and the Victoria's Secret catalogue, Tyra had to be confident in taking on the established standards for a model and challenging them, or she would have never accomplished what she did (and make history in the process).

I've had the pleasure of photographing Tyra on a number of occasions. She comes to the set calm, composed, prepared, and ready to work. She has innate talent in front of the camera that's hard to parallel. But what makes her especially good at what she does is her confidence. She knows she has what the shoot requires, so she delivers the goods, time after time.

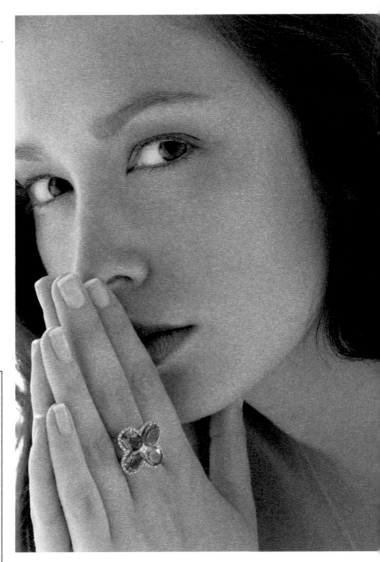

Kaiulani Swan

Confidence is one of the most attractive qualities of inner beauty, but it has to be in the right proportion. Overconfidence can make you appear stupid, giddy, or worse still, conceited. There is a fine line between confidence and conceit. You don't ever want to be accused of appearing superior, flaunting your success, or acting like you know it all. Being confident doesn't mean showing off; it means knowing that you have the ability to do something without needing to broadcast it.

Conversely, in your life's "auditions," you certainly *want* to convey that you want the job (you do, don't you?). I've had girls come in to go-sees who act so nonchalant about being there that they hardly even say hello, shake your hand, or look you in the eye—yet you know they waited an hour to see you, in a room with a hundred other girls! What they are doing is *feigning* confidence, but, unfortunately, an "I don't need this" attitude can come off even more arrogant than loud overconfidence can.

I am certainly not expecting a girl who is eager for a potential opportunity to come bounding in like a puppy dog, wagging her tail. No amount of unfounded confidence can ever magically bring about sudden talent. But standing tall, making eye contact, and showing good manners go a long way toward leaving a memorable impression of yourself, wherever you go.

SOMETIMES BAD GIRLS ARE GOOD (MODELS)

I'll admit, sometimes a conceited, rude girl can photograph really well. Perhaps it's the self-confidence she has from knowing her ability in front of the camera that causes her to act like she has it all. But know this: I never rebook anyone who has shown herself to be more trouble than she is worth or caused the whole job to be a drag.

Confidence can get you in the door. But if you want to be invited back, use that confidence to show you are a team player.

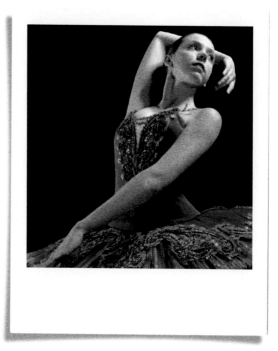

PROFILE IN CONFIDENCE

KATIE BOREN

"Confidence is the most important personality trait for inner beauty. If you are not confident with yourself and who you are on the inside, then you will never feel truly beautiful. Besides, if you don't view yourself as truly beautiful, then no one else will."

Katie Boren, an accomplished ballerina who hails from Dallas, Texas, has been dancing since she was three years old. At the ripe old age of eleven, Katie landed her first gig with the American Ballet Theater (ABT). She has since become part of the professional dance company ABT II. Do you want to know what she thinks is the secret to her success? Confidence!

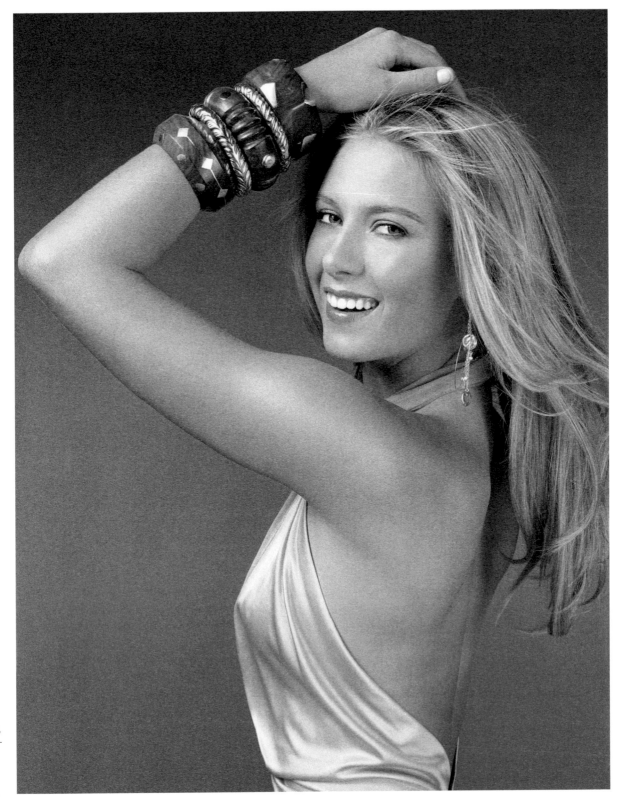

One of the chief suggestions I give young models when trying to help them connect with their confidence and pride—the kind that's deserved and earned, not imagined and faked—is that they do this simple yet highly effective exercise:

Imagine you have won an Olympic medal. The gold! Think about the years of training it has taken. The sweat and hard work you've put in leading up to this monumental moment. The eyes of the entire world are on you in anticipation of your response. Because you (yes, you!) have outshone the competition with your stellar performance. You now stand on the podium as a beacon of light, representing the best of the best, while being broadcast all over the globe and to galaxies far, far away.

Now, if you literally try to picture yourself in that scene, you automatically start to stand up tall, straightening your shoulders, elongating your neck, and radiating pride. When I do the exercise, the hair on the back of my neck stands on end and I get goose bumps (but that's just me). Imagine your national anthem playing in the background as your country's flag is being raised, your eyes almost tearing, but beaming all the while. Snap!—that's the shot!

Of course, if you're feeling that you've won simply because you're better than everyone else, you've missed the point completely. That arrogance will read in your eyes, and you will appear far from beautiful. In fact, conceit is one of the ugliest emotions you can have, and no matter how pretty your facade may be, that inner ugliness will shine through every time.

CONFIDENCE IN VOGUE

TOCCARA JONES

"I'm big, black, beautiful, and lovin' it."

One girl who embodies confidence in just the right way is the unforgettable Toccara Jones. In addition to her outer beauty, she is charming and lively, and she always startles and enchants with her ability to "tell it like it is." She is able to walk into a room and inspire you with her self-confidence. She knows she has a sense of humor and she uses it: "Every man wants some meat on his girl's bones. Ain't nobody want a bone except a dog, and they bury them." She has been labeled a "plus-size" model and she owns her figure, presenting herself with such comfort and pride that she makes you love it too.

Although she can be brutally honest, she always has modesty and a heart. Her confidence never turns into conceit. And she always tempers her confidence with gratitude and common sense. She'd never belittle a competitor, but neither would she miss out on an opportunity. And, often to endearingly comic effect, she never quashes a chance to succeed due to false modesty.

Toccara makes a lasting impression. People ask after her regularly, and I am always glad to report that she continues on with an impressive career. (Did you know that Toccara was the first ANTM "graduate" to be featured in Vogue, photographed by the legendary Steven Meisel, for Italian Vogue?)

Maria Sharapova

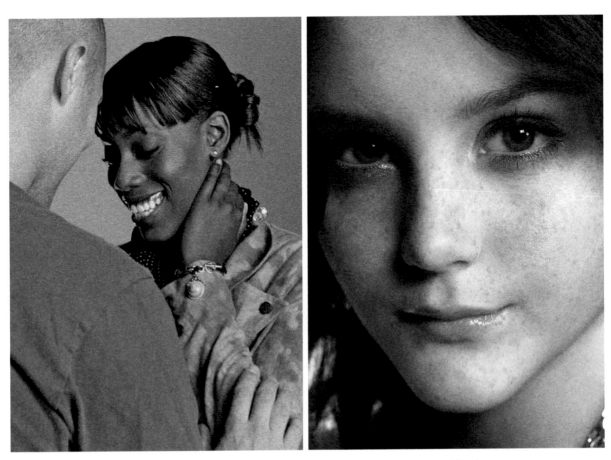

Working with the Make-A-Wish Foundation to fulfill the wishes of Mercedes Andrews (left) and Madeline Finnegan (right) to become a supermodel for a day

A FINAL WORD— A GIFT FROM TRUE BEAUTIES

I have worked for many years as a wish granter for the Make-A-Wish Foundation, and the young women I've photographed in that capacity have been some of the most beautiful ever to grace my lens. Girls with life-threatening illnesses, who have risen above it all in the pursuit of one thing: life. Working to get a beauty shot takes a lot of courage on their behalf. Finding their beauty, on the other hand, was possibly one of the easiest assignments I've ever had, and an honor for me.

These young Make-A-Wish girls, whose wish I was meant to be granting by making them supermodels for a day, inadvertently granted me a wish. They showed me that real confidence and courage is pure and unpretentious. A given right for all of us, if we shed our useless insecurities, realize that everything we are looking for is right at our fingertips, and believe in ourselves.

1. "DEAR FUTURE SELF"

The biggest enemy of self-confidence is that little voice inside our heads that tells us we're not good enough, tall enough, this enough, that enough. Let's kill any negative inner voices inside of you. Pick your weapon of choice and annihilate that nasty little demon. Good riddance! Now that it's gone, you are free to stop saying, "I'm no good at that," and start saying, "I'm going to get better at that."

Reference the lists you made from the Casting Call writing assignment, the physical and emotional attributes that are unique and wonderful about you. Now, accentuate the positive! Fashion these lists of attributes into a short letter to your future self. Make it fun, affirm all your best qualities, and explain to yourself why you deserve to be confident in any situation. Maybe you need to give yourself a pep talk or maybe you just need a friendly reminder. Add this to your portfolio and read it every morning. Start the day knowing you are working toward being fierce and afraid of nothing! Write!

2. YOUR GOLDEN MOMENT

Remember the exercise I described earlier in this chapter, where models envision the moment they win a gold medal at the Olympics? It's time for you to try it. First, make it real. What is your sport and what country do you represent?

Next, set up your camera, leaving it poised for you to set off the autotimer when you're good and ready. Imagine that's the TV crew that's going to beam your image into homes all over the world. Stand on your "podium" and listen to your country's national anthem coming over the loudspeakers—or better yet, blast your "confidence theme song." Hit that autotimer, get back into position, and really feel it. You have reached this moment through hours of hard work, overcoming all obstacles in your way. It is a moment of supreme pride. Flash! There goes your gold-medal self-portrait!

Dear Future Self,

Good morning! Here are five things I want you to remember today and every day:

1. *You have a pretty smile and people respond to it.*
2. *You're an excellent volleyball player, because you know how to go for it in the clutch.*
3. *You look best when you hold your shoulders back and stand tall — even when it makes you feel too tall (you're not).*
4. *You've got strong arms and shapely legs, and there's nothing wrong with flaunting it.*
5. *You have an amazing family who loves you, so you must be extremely lovable!*

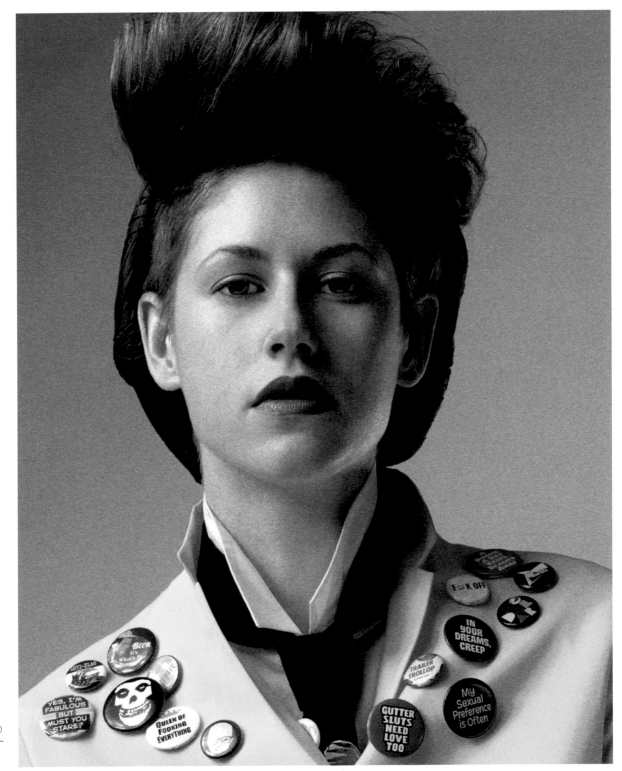

ANTM contestant Shandi Sullivan, fearlessly taking on the Fear Factor challenge

Isolate something that scares you. Is it doing karaoke in front of a crowd of strangers? Is it that mangy growling dog down the street? Or the horror film you saw on Halloween? Once you pick something, try to deduce what about it makes you afraid. Think back on a moment of weakness you had in the face of this thing.

Now, I am empowering you. You are a superwoman! You have all the control and the confidence you need to stand up and squash this thing.

Get your camera ready and look straight over the lens. Something just beyond that camera is the fear you despise. Doesn't look so bad at the moment (looks like a camera), but tap into the confidence inside yourself and stare past that camera with your most courageous look. Throw your fists in the air if you have to. Knock your fear right out with a one-two punch! You have the power now. Take a self-portrait!

Eye contact is of the utmost importance when it comes to demonstrating your confidence. Confident eyes are not mean or vengeful eyes; confident eyes are eyes filled with sparkle, intelligence, and grace. Think about people who speak to you with their eyes as well as their voices: Oprah Winfrey, President Obama . . . think about Tyra during eliminations on *ANTM*. Her eyes never wander, and she never conveys that someone's a failure or that she thinks she's better than them. She is confidently speaking the results of the panel.

Usually, in taking a beauty shot, you want to pretend you are looking at someone way out beyond the lens. But this time, make eye contact with your camera. You love that camera. You are not scared of that camera. But neither are you superior to that camera. You are proud of yourself and radiating your confidence with your eyes alone. Take a self-portrait!

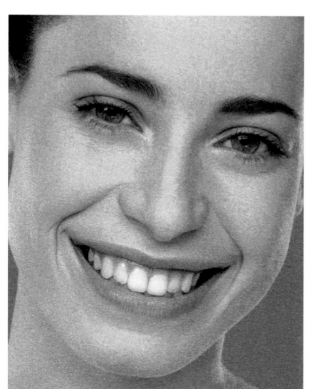

Yuliya Malamud, twenty, student, capturing confidence

NOW, as you add these self-portraits to your portfolio, who do you see? Is she confident and ready for the next element of the Beauty Equation? Is she fierce? I think she is.

Remember, as you go forward into the next chapter, that confidence is key, but courage is equally essential. Having courage doesn't mean you know you can do something; it means you're willing to give it your best shot. Bravery is a powerful, hypnotic trait of beauty that wins hearts and minds. Whether you win or not, you can be proud of your efforts and, from that strength, build confidence.

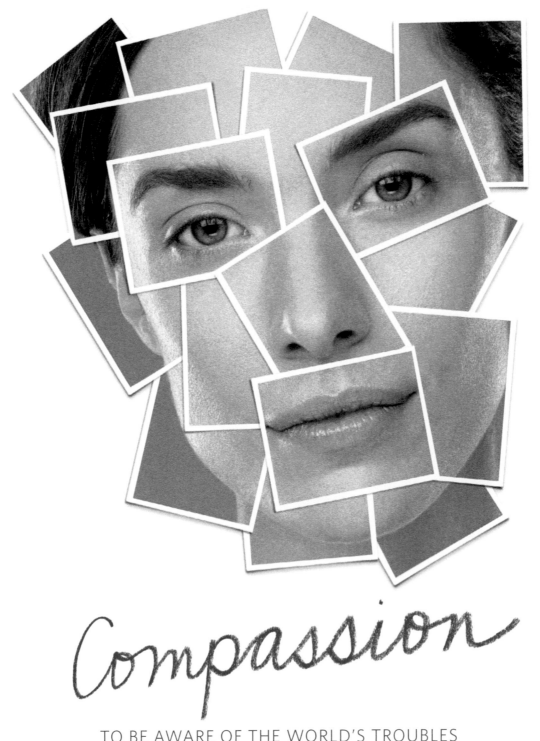

Compassion

TO BE AWARE OF THE WORLD'S TROUBLES
AND DO SOMETHING ABOUT IT

"Be kind whenever possible. It is always possible."

—Dalai Lama

Model Citizen: *the teach*

LEARNING FROM OUR ELDERS

I want you to take a moment and think about your grandmother or a woman who has been like a grandmother to you. Picture her in your head. Would you describe her as beautiful? Without hesitation, I think most people would respond with an enthusiastic, "Of course!"

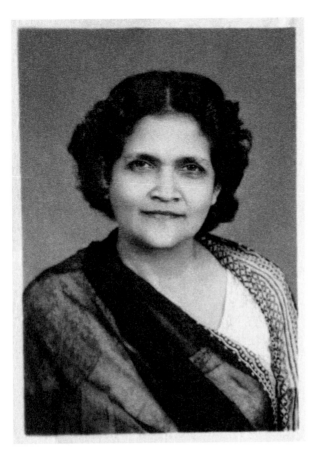

My grandmother, Ines Thorne

"From what we get, we can make a living; what we give, however, makes a life."

—Arthur Ashe, tennis pro

I'm not talking about putting her in six-inch heels and a designer frock and sending her down the runway in Milan. In fact, her appearance doesn't actually matter that much. She is beautiful because you see her as such. And that very likely stems from your lifelong relationship with her, a woman who always took care of you. A woman who always knew when you were coming down with a cold and had just the remedy to make you feel better. A woman who could recognize when you had your feelings hurt and needed a hug. A woman who couldn't resist seeing your joy when spoiling you with the ice cream or presents your parents wouldn't allow. The paragon of compassion. She was always highly aware of your needs and instinctually did anything in her power to make you better, happier, more safe and secure.

Now let's talk about you. Compassion begins with you and ends with someone else. We've often heard the advice "Until you learn to love yourself, it is impossible for you to love anyone else." I believe this is true. But loving yourself is quite different from loving something or someone else. It's not like the love you have for a precious piece of jewelry or your favorite movie star because of the happiness they bring you. Loving yourself doesn't mean "me first!" or "my needs above all others, dammit!"

Put another way, you can't use yourself as the *object* of your love. Self-love comes from within. It's about knowing who you are while accurately perceiving what is going on around you so that you effortlessly project the most beautiful you. I'm going to show you the way to find this for yourself—paradoxically, through love for others. Compassion. It's one of the key elements of the Beauty Equation.

"Someone who is both successful and humble is a rare and truly beautiful combination."

—Amber Kallor, beauty assistant, *Glamour*

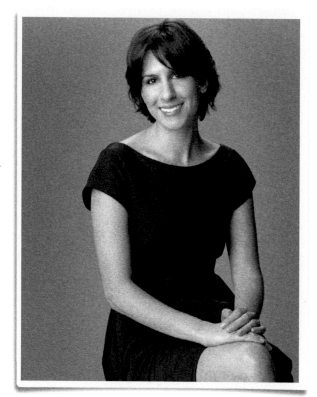

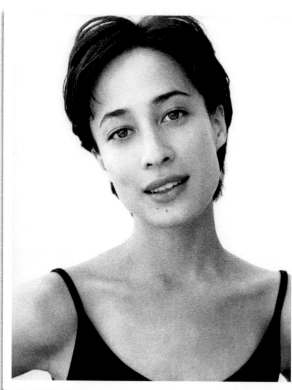

"Maybe if we spent the same amount of time and money helping other people feel beautiful as we do on ourselves, the world would be a better place."

—Kimmy Hise, Crissy Barker's twin sister

"I have a very clear memory of being in nursery school and being taught the Golden Rule: 'Do unto others as you would have them do unto you.' Compassion to me is internalizing the feelings of others and relating your own life to the world around you. The Golden Rule begins with *Do*—a call to action. Treat others with compassion and when you feel their pain and struggle, do all you can to help them."

—Crissy Barker

IN THE BEGINNING

When I was a kid in London, my family got me off to a great start in understanding compassion. I grew up spending holidays with my family, but not always at home around the Christmas tree or hunting down Easter eggs on the lawn. My parents would sometimes round up my brothers, sisters, and me, and, instead of giving us presents or baskets filled with candy, they'd take us down to the homeless shelter, where we would all volunteer our services in the soup kitchen or whip up some cookie dough for a bake sale to raise money for the local community. It might sound like work, but it wasn't. It was a lot of fun.

Both of my parents were instrumental in teaching me how self-empowering it is to give back. It's something that I've carried with me my entire life and that I'm very grateful for. "The pleasure is in the giving, not the receiving," they say.

Still, keeping it real, it would be a serious drag to not have a present waiting for you on Christmas Day or during Hanukkah. There's nothing wrong with accepting a gift, compliment, or reward. On the contrary, it's wonderful. But sometimes the greatest gift, compliment, or reward is written on the face of someone you have helped. Offer a bowl of hot soup to a hungry homeless person on a cold day and you'll see what I mean.

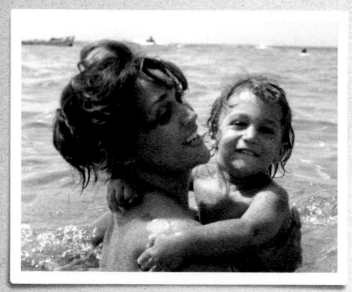

My mom and me swimming off the coast of
Sanotorino, Greece.

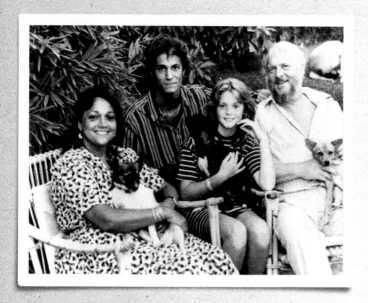

My mother, me (age 15), my sister, Mary-Anne,
and my father.

Me (age 9) and my sister, Mary-Anne.

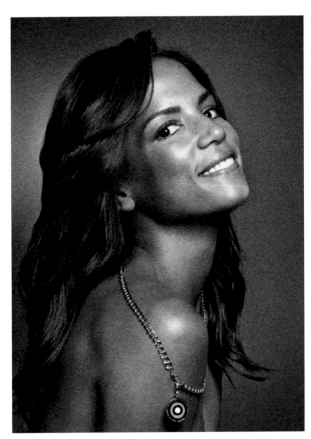
Model, actress, and friend Veronica Webb and I, teaming up to shoot a campaign for Fashion Targets Breast Cancer

LUCKY ME

Please don't take all this as me anointing myself Saint Barker! I am one incredibly lucky man—but I've capitalized on that luck by grabbing opportunity by the horns each time it came my way. Then, once I'm dealt a winning hand, my first instinct is to parlay that hand into as much as I can for everyone around me. Now more than ever, as the father of two young and impressionable little people, I try to set an example that will inspire. I don't ever want to be the kind of father who just tells his kids what to do and what to think. I want them to look up to their dad as a guy who acts on his word, and to love themselves enough to have faith in their own decisions.

A friend of mine once had a summer job working in a restaurant. There were two managers. One was great and the other was, in everyone's honest assessment, a real twit. Everyone dreaded working a shift with the bad manager who, at the end of the day, when everything had to be broken down and thoroughly scrubbed and cleaned, would sit with his feet up and just bark orders. The good manager, on the other hand, would roll up her sleeves and dig right into the dirty work, not even asking the employees "below her" to help.

When the bad manager made such demands, my friend and his coworkers resented their work, and a very destructive negativity would develop. When people saw the good manager's enthusiasm at being a peer and not their "superior," on the other hand, what do you think the employees did? They jumped right in, with a smile—and ended up doing a better overall job. And my friend carried the good manager in his heart as an example to emulate ever since. It's the reverse of the often repeated parental fallback "Do as I say, not as I do." If you want to set an example, be that example. Don't just bark out what the example should be. You are bound to lose the popularity contest of life and go home empty-handed and empty-hearted.

KEEP IT CLOSE TO HOME: USE WHAT *YOU* DO TO HELP OTHERS

What do you have to offer? Can you sing or play an instrument? Perform at a retirement home; many welcome entertainment with enthusiasm. Do you have a flair for writing? Craft an article about something or someone that needs attention and submit it to your local newspaper. Are you are a wiz at Web design? Offer your services to a local nonprofit organization, like a pet rescue or a school. Everyone has some talent that could be put to use helping others. All it takes is a little creativity and the desire to lend a hand.

In recent years I have begun making documentary films. Inspired by the selfless work of many amazing people I've come to know, I wanted to share how these compassionate folks concern themselves with the suffering of others and have the will and determination to do something about it. I know I am always enthused when I watch a documentary film about someone who has changed the world through their incredible work, and I saw this undertaking as a natural progression from my photography. When people congratulate me for sharing the stories of these dedicated souls, it brings a smile to my face, because I feel that my documentaries congratulate the people who are truly doing the good work.

HAITI

HUNGER AND HOPE

As the poorest country in the Western Hemisphere, Haiti was in dire straits even before being hit by one of the worst earthquakes in modern history. Before the quake hit, I traveled with my team to Cité Soleil, one of the most impoverished neighborhoods in Port-au-Prince, the capital of Haiti. We were scheduled to arrive after a series of riots over food shortages. The U.S. Embassy had temporarily closed, warning that if we went there, it could not guarantee our safety. After much debate, we decided to go anyway, as we knew that the prevailing situation only meant the people there needed us all the more. Their story had to be told.

It would have been more convenient, of course, to postpone the trip and ignore the situation, hoping someone else would help, but that would have been the easy road. The trip turned out to be one of the most moving experiences of our lives. We saw that, despite the hunger and tumult, there was hope.

We saw young men and women doing all they possibly could, under extremely adverse conditions, to support not just their own families but also complete strangers. We witnessed selfless acts by old and young alike. Our mere presence made those we met feel acknowledged, like somebody in the world cared, and we were widely welcomed with open arms.

The resulting film and photographs were hauntingly beautiful, but what I personally walked away with was a renewed sense of compassion for humankind. I learned that we need to love one another in order to bring love to ourselves.

To that end, I am now a board member of the Haitian charity Edeyo (which translates to "help them" in Haitian Creole) and do all I can to keep Haiti and its people in the public eye.

(DOWNLOAD)

SONGS THAT CHANGED THE WORLD

*"You may say I'm a dreamer,
but I'm not the only one.
I hope someday you'll join us,
and the world will live as one."*

"Imagine" —JOHN LENNON

"We Are the World" —USA FOR AFRICA

"We Are the World 25 for Haiti" —ARTISTS FOR HAITI

"Free Nelson Mandela" —THE SPECIAL A.K.A.

"Sun City" —ARTISTS UNITED AGAINST APARTHEID

"Do They Know It's Christmas?" —BAND AID

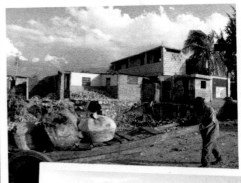

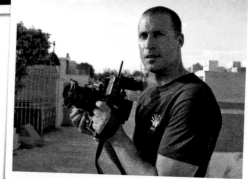

Filming my documentary *Haiti: Hunger and Hope*

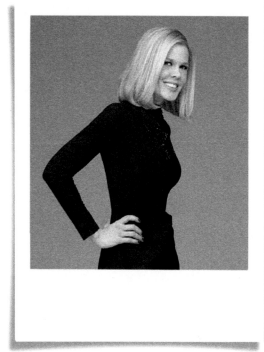

Fashion stylist and expert, and national fashion ambassador for the Make-A-Wish Foundation

WISH-GRANTING GENIE

MARY ALICE STEPHENSON

"The Make-A-Wish teenagers I work with have battled life-threatening illnesses bravely and have had, in many cases, to put their dreams on hold. It is not only an honor but my mission to work with our industry to make sure that every one of these [kids'] fashion wishes are granted and that these kids get to experience the joy and healing power of having a dream come true. I hope to compel people of all ages to help others achieve their dreams as they are striving to realize their own. When you've experienced the impact of granting a wish firsthand, it is not only inspirational, it's life-changing!"

"Money is like manure; it's not worth a thing unless it's spread around encouraging young things to grow." —Thornton Wilder

IT'S NICE TO BE NICE TO THE NICE

I know it might sound trite, but one person really can make a difference. Over the years, I have met and photographed so many extraordinary people who have dedicated their lives to helping those in need. People who, through their celebrity or ingenuity (and always their passion), have often raised millions of dollars to effect change, right wrongs, and make the world a better place. And remember, every little bit counts.

And while money helps, it's not the only way to be charitable. Individuals with big ideas but small bank accounts have done wonders in the name of goodwill, and so can you. For inspiration, take a look at the CNN Heroes ("Everyday People Changing the World") Web site (www.cnn.com/SPECIALS/cnn.heroes/) to find dozens of stories about people of modest means who have tapped into community resources to improve people's lives, at home and around the globe.

Over the past couple of years, in my work with the Make-A-Wish Foundation, we have granted more than twenty wishes with the help of Oprah Winfrey, Mary Alice Stephenson, and a multitude of fashion giants. We've helped young girls who—despite all the hardship, pain, and worry they and their young bodies have gone through—simply wish to feel like a model, if only for a day. And just like any young girl, you can imagine the confidence it gives them to be pampered and fawned over by professional makeup artists and hair stylists, and then brought center stage under the lights and my lens. As for us seasoned fashion pros, helping these girls feel a connection to their inner glow is its own reward.

Supermodel Gisele Bündchen surprises Amanda Acala on the set of her Make-A-Wish photo shoot

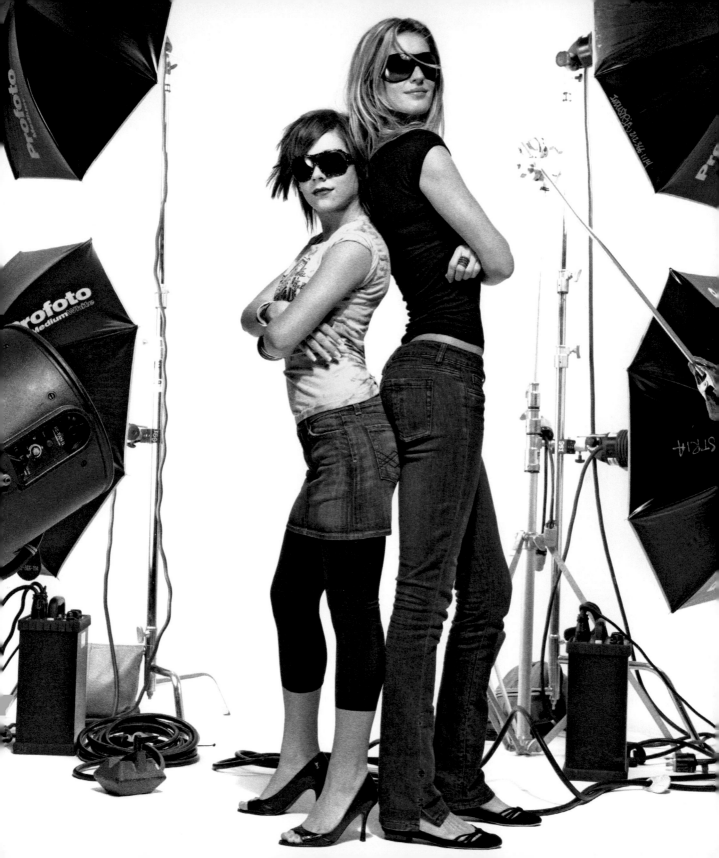

Among the girls I shot for the Make-A-Wish Foundation was Destanee Clark. Destanee passed away while I was writing this book, driving home harder than ever the importance of doing the right thing whenever you can. I'll never forget the brightness Destanee brought to the set. Her star will always shine in my heart.

We also shot an advertising campaign for the foundation empowering everyone to be a wish granter. The point was simple: Celebrities are great inspirations, but you don't need to be rich or famous (or capable of performing magic) to grant somebody a wish. You just need to be there, listen, and understand. Surely, if magic exists at all, it's when someone feels their wish has been granted even before they realized what it was.

Perform simple acts of kindness: That's all it takes. Volunteer your time to pick a recent widow or widower up and take them to the movies, cook a warm dinner for an elderly neighbor, help a friend dig the car out of the driveway in a snowstorm—and, above all else, take the time to actually listen to people.

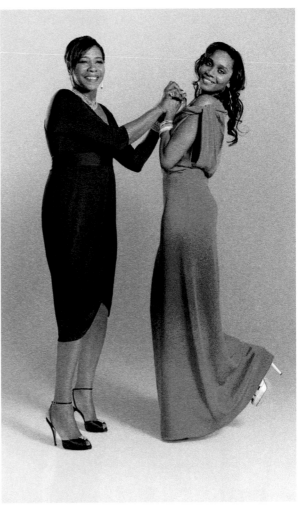

Destanee Clark and her mother, whom I shot for the Make-A-Wish Foundation (the photo appeared in *O, the Oprah Magazine*)

"My 6-iron has the power to grant a wish."

Golf is my life. But the Make-A-Wish Foundation® helped me see that it's much more. Many children with life-threatening medical conditions wish they could tee it up at a famous course. Or meet their favorite golfers. The PGA TOUR and LPGA help in every way imaginable. I said, "sign me up! I want to play in that game."
We all have the power to grant a wish. Start your journey with Destination Joy™ at Wish.org

MAKE (A) WISH.
SHARE THE POWER OF A WISH.

Annika Sörenstam for the Make-A-Wish Foundation

So you see what I'm getting at. When you go out of your way for someone, you always get a greater return on your investment. Compassion comes in all shapes and sizes. It doesn't always have to come from someone famous, with a lot of money. It doesn't even have to involve a serious cause. It can be as simple as opening the door for someone, a polite gesture, picking up the disposable coffee cup you find on the nature trail and putting it where it belongs. All these little things add up.

People will usually respond immediately to kindness. They'll smile and give you a friendly "thank you" in return. Your friends and family will notice your selfless acts too, and will hold you in higher esteem and be inspired by you. But the greatest reward of compassion doesn't come from others; it comes from inside. It's the simple satisfaction of knowing you've done the right thing.

Showing common courtesy, leading by example, having an open heart, and actively going out of your way to help others is single-handedly the easiest way to build your own sense of worth, which will naturally build your confidence (which we know adds to your Beauty Equation). And talk about allure! A feeling of self-worth communicates a special, modest confidence, the kind that might serve you someday when you find yourself walking quietly into a loud room where others are gathered in your honor, whispering "thank you," and causing a hush to fall, as those around you are humbled by your presence. Think I'm exaggerating? Consider the awe and respect we all share for leaders known for their compassion: Gandhi, Mother Teresa, Nelson Mandela.

It might seem arrogant, imagining all this coming your way just because you're lending a helping hand. But show me the harm in striving to be better and to make a better world in order to build your own sense of pride, and to be able to hold your head up high, and truly glow from within.

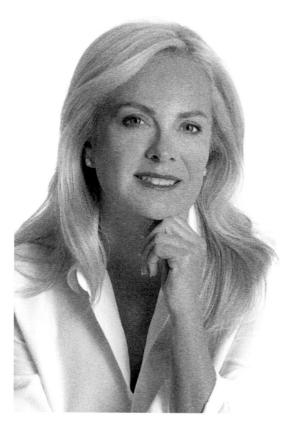

"Inner beauty is putting others before you. From the minute they could speak, I taught my children to be courteous and polite to others. As they grew, people would always tell me that my children were polite and that they were beautiful inside and out. That is such a huge compliment to me as a parent. It means much more to me than being a designer."

—Pamella DeVos, designer of Pamella Roland

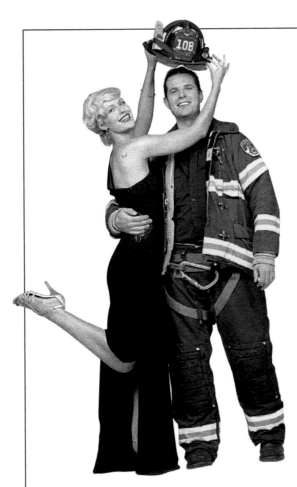

ANTM winner Caridee English with her brother, New York firefighter Scott Specht

PROFILE IN COMPASSION

CARIDEE ENGLISH

"My big brother was always a hero in my eyes. I wanted to be just like him and looked up to him. His constant bravery and courage paved a path for me to [show] the same. We have two very different jobs, but we both beat the odds, and every day has its new challenges. He protects me, and I encourage him."

Caridee is one of the most charismatic girls you'll ever meet. As lovely as she is, she suffers from psoriasis, a chronic, non-contagious disease that causes red, scaly patches on the skin. Despite this hurdle, she's ridden a wave of success all the way to a thriving career in fashion and music (gorgeous Caridee plays drums in a rock band). She is very open about the disease and actively dispels rumors as to what it isn't. She has publicly stated that when she was young, she felt "cursed" by her affliction, and that she had been taunted her whole life because people thought it was contagious.

"Psoriasis awareness is very important to me. I want others with the disease to know they are not alone. I want to inspire them to live their dreams," says Caridee.

Caridee decided to make her "curse" her cause. With her star rising, she has become a spokesperson for the National Psoriasis Foundation, spreading awareness and encouraging others to seek treatment. She has given selflessly to help others, partly inspired by her firefighter brother. She has also donated her time in the fights for animal rights, toward legalizing gay marriage, and has worked with me at the Make-A-Wish Foundation. Caridee is a true beauty—and doesn't knowing all this about her make her seem even more stunning?

TOP TO BOTTOM
Caridee English with Ramona Goodall, for the Make-A-Wish Foundation

Caridee English with Emily Rawley, for the Make-A-Wish Foundation

Caridee English with Gabriela Bonicichi, for the Make-A-Wish Foundation

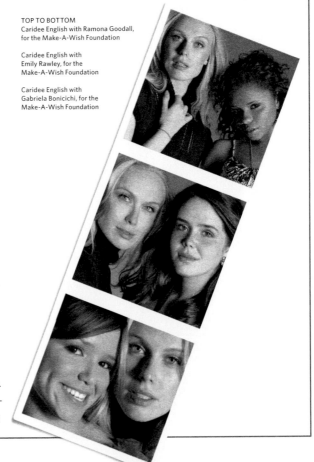

NO GOOD DEED GOES UNPUNISHED

The Dalai Lama said, "If you want others to be happy, practice compassion. If you want to be happy, practice compassion." And ultimately, for most of us, happiness is the goal of life.

Of course, you cannot always expect to be thanked or acknowledged for the good things you do. In fact, don't be surprised if sometimes you get your hand slapped, a grimace of ingratitude, or even the finger. But so what?

Not all people can handle compassion. How many times have you let someone cut in front of you on the freeway, held the door for someone and received no thanks, or wished a stranger a good morning and received no response? It happens all the time, and makes you wonder what's so difficult about making the little effort it takes to be courteous or respond. I see these "haters" as not loving themselves. They are giving themselves the bum's rush and can't help but dole it out to everyone around them in their campaigns to make the world a lousier place. But that's where you have to embrace that you are right and they are wrong—and that particular brand of righteousness is well placed when you've acted with your heart. No matter what reaction you experience, know this: Being indifferent to the problems around you does *nothing* for your quest to be a more beautiful person and live in a better world. So don't ever feel discouraged. Just chalk any negativity you encounter up in the "oh, well" column and keep at it!

Quick List

Things We Learned in Grade School That Still Go a Long Way

"Consideration for others is the basis of a good life, a good society." —Confucius

1. Smile
2. Say please and thank-you
3. Pay someone a compliment
4. Hold the door for someone
5. Do a funny dance (make someone laugh)

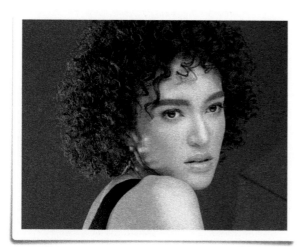

"I have always had a deep sense of compassion for others, especially young women like myself. In order to pursue my dreams the way I wanted, I had to push aside negative self-images and learn compassion, forgiveness, and belief within myself. There I found confidence, courage, and beauty."

—*ANTM* winner Naima Mora

"A human being is a part of the whole called by us 'universe,' a part limited in time and space. He experiences himself, his thoughts, and feelings as something separated from the rest, a kind of optical delusion of his consciousness. This delusion is a kind of prison for us, restricting us to our personal desires and to affection for a few persons nearest to us. Our task must be to free ourselves from this prison by widening our circle of compassion to embrace all living creatures and the whole of nature in its beauty."

—Albert Einstein

Another organization I am involved with is the Humane Society of the United States. I am the spokesperson for their Protect Seals campaign; I feel very strongly about looking out for animals, not just people. We all share this planet and if we are to hold our heads up high, we need to treat every living thing with compassion and humanity.

In my work, I have been lucky enough to travel to eastern Canada to witness the birth of harp seals, who start life off as fluffy little white coats and quickly mature into mottled silvery steel creatures. One of the things I documented up on the ice was how similar to humans the mother seals behaved with their young, and how precocious and childlike (even like my own children) the seal pups were.

Whether you eat meat is not the issue. Making educated decisions about how we behave and how we treat animals and people around us is. We can't expect to have a happier and healthier world unless we nurture it and know that, when we hurt the planet, we hurt ourselves. You may think that helping one animal or one person makes no difference in the grand scheme of things, but it makes a difference to them. And that's beautiful.

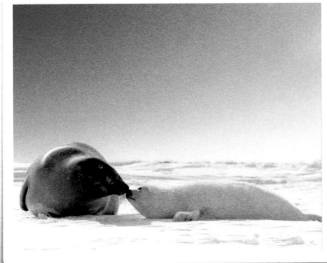

While filming my documentary *A Sealed Fate?*

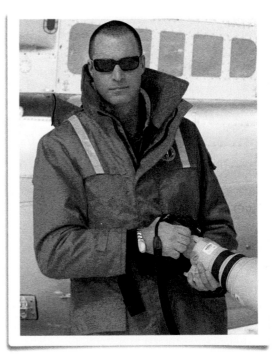

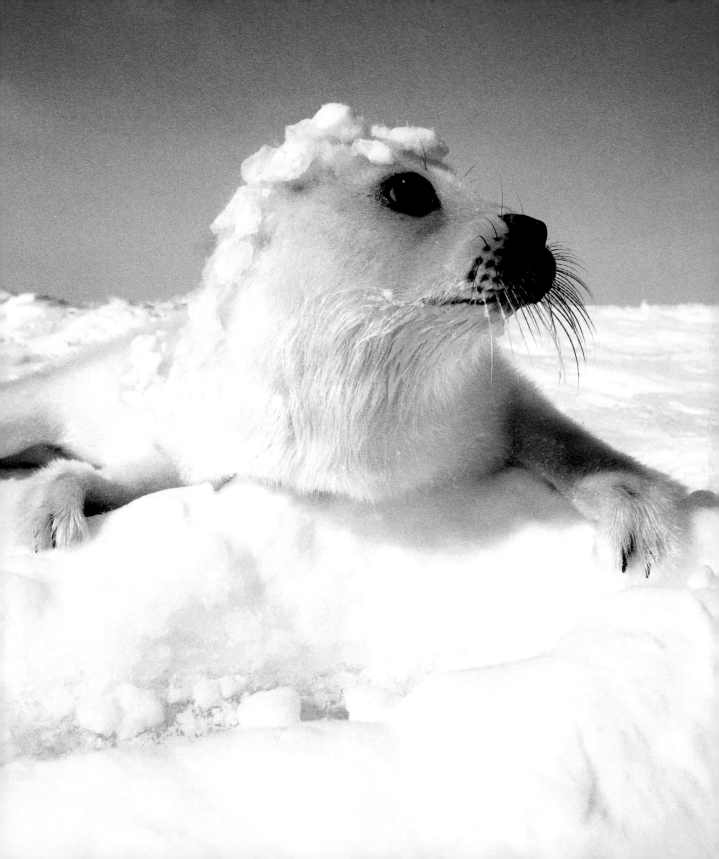

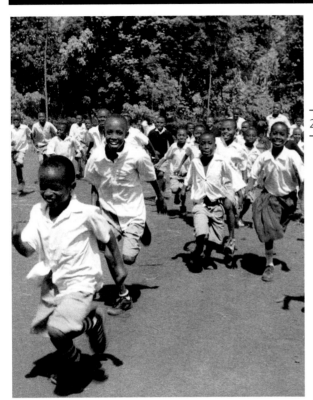

In Tanzania, on a mission to stop the spread of pediatric AIDS

1. IF I COULD CHANGE THE WORLD

Think about the things in your world that bother you. What people or situations do you feel could be better if only they had a little tender loving care? What things close to home could be improved? Is there a nearby park that needs some trees and vegetation? Is there an elderly person down the street who is all alone and rarely gets visitors? Is your father having trouble making ends meet?

Try to isolate five things you think need help in your world. If there's a larger national or global problem, that's great too. Just concentrate on what you would like to change if you could. Now, record these in your portfolio. Write!

PS: I'm not going to ask you to run out and attend to these concerns immediately. But when you are done, I do want you to research the things you care about. Are there already organizations doing something about them? Can you help out in any way? Volunteer? Over the next year, think about your list and make a concerted effort to help.

2. FEEL THE LOVE

Think about someone close to you who you think of as caring very passionately about you. Is it your mother? A teacher? Your best friend? It can be anyone in your life, just make it someone who you feel always has your back—someone who knows when you are in need and, even without you asking, does something about it.

Now get your camera ready, and try to channel this person. They have great love for you, and now you're going to feel what they feel inside. For this moment, try to love yourself the way someone else does. Look toward the camera through their eyes and imagine the camera is you. Take a self-portrait!

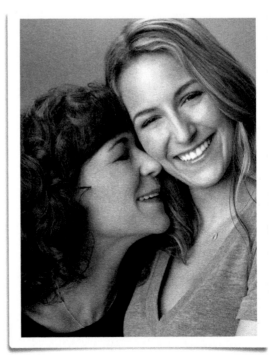

April Franzino, assistant beauty editor, *Good Housekeeping*, with her mother, Debbie Franzino

Now I want you to isolate one of the five things you came up with in the writing exercise. Pick the one thing closest to your heart that you feel needs help. Needs *your* help.

Now, as you think about this thing, letting it touch your heart, truly feel your desire to help, to make a difference, to affect the situation. Maybe thinking about it makes you feel hopeless, because the situation as it stands is overwhelming; maybe it makes you feel angry, because you want to take action right now; or maybe it makes you feel sad, because you suddenly identify with someone else's pain. Whatever your reaction, set up your camera and show me through your eyes the compassion you have. Take a self-portrait!

For your final self-portrait in this chapter, I want you to visualize change. Imagine the thing you have perceived as needing help. Now imagine what you would (and probably will someday) do to make that thing right. Imagine the comfort or joy or benefits your actions will have brought about. Feel the warm rays of knowing you've made a difference. The world is a better place because of you. Take a self-portrait!

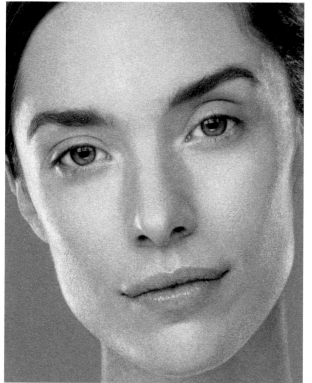

ALTHOUGH we cannot and should not expect praise and adulation for being charitable, we can and we should feel good about ourselves for stepping up when the opportunity arises. And one thing's for certain: The opportunities abound. Make yourself feel more beautiful by going out and finding one today—right now!

Lauren Cotton, twenty-six, professional nanny, capturing compassion

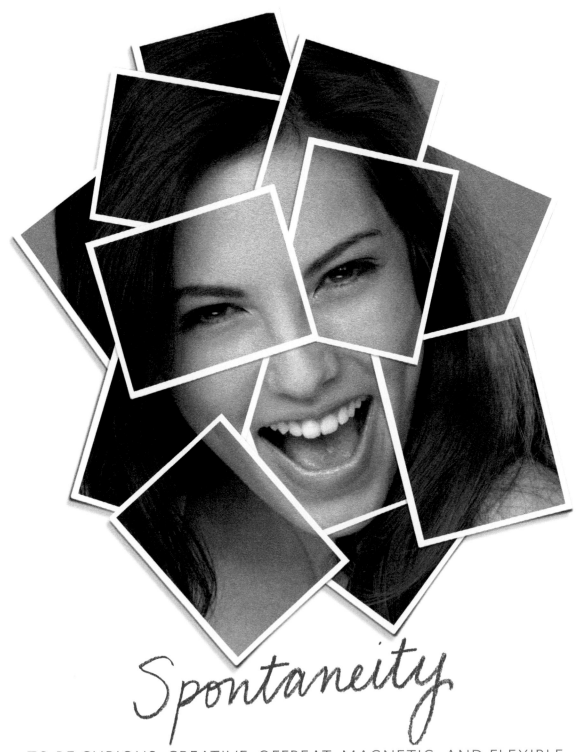

Spontaneity

TO BE CURIOUS, CREATIVE, OFFBEAT, MAGNETIC, AND FLEXIBLE

> "Our spontaneous action is always the best. You cannot, with your best deliberation and heed, come so close to any question as your spontaneous glance shall bring you."
>
> —Ralph Waldo Emerson

Natural Chemistry: *the teach*

A DAY TO REMEMBER

I remember the day I met my wife, Crissy. I walked into our modeling agency in Milan and there she was, sitting on a bench, waiting to speak to an agent. She had just arrived from the United States and was full of anticipation. I immediately approached her and, not knowing what to say but knowing I wanted to say something, blurted out that I had an impressive collection of mosquito bites on my arm. Not my finest pickup line, but it came out of my mouth spontaneously, and Crissy responded with care and curiosity.

Funny thing was, she wasn't flirtatious, nor forward in any manner, which only made me more fascinated and determined to get to know her—and hopefully explain there was more to me than unsightly red bumps on my arms. Crissy had always been a free spirit who never judged a book by its cover, but it took me months to so much as get her to agree to go out on a date! She played hard to get, showing me that, to be right for her, I needed to demonstrate patience, dedication, and loyalty—all of which has led to our being together ever since. And it was all thanks to that first spontaneous hello.

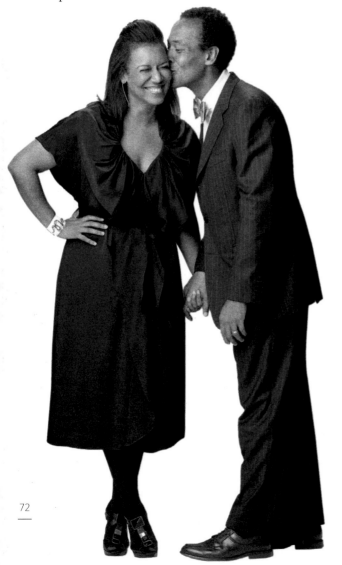

DO THE MATH!

Bet you didn't know this: As a teenager, I studied biology, chemistry, physics, and mathematics! So you can trust me when I tell you that chemistry is not just that certain something between two people. It's the science of things coming together—atoms, molecules, matter—inside of you and out in the world, and the very natural way in which they create spontaneous reactions with each other.

At this point in the Beauty Equation, you have been working on "adding" elements to yourself: allure, confidence, compassion. As those new elements swirl about within, you are having new experiences, new feelings, and finding new energy. Chemistry is all about the changes that occur when you bring elemental forces up against one another. The pot begins to boil, the reaction takes hold . . . and pow! Something seemingly spontaneous occurs. Ironically, that's the science of it—it isn't spontaneous at all. It's expected. Add things together and something happens.

It should be happening to you right now. Let it out! It should feel great.

Spontaneity is the essence of personal pleasure, not only because it makes you feel free, but because it is the culmination of an inner development that is allowing that freedom. Make your head spin? Good! On the one hand, it's a mathematical equation: The more you develop, the freer you feel. On the other, it feels like a total mystery: What will you do next? Nobody knows, not even you.

And it's the reverse of scary. It's exhilarating. Exciting. Like falling in love. Or better yet, like falling in love with life, exactly as it is, exactly as it comes to you, in the moment.

"The journey of life is as important as the numerous destinations."

—Pam Edwards Christiani, style and beauty editor, *People*, with her husband, Nigel Christiani

Crissy Barker and her sister, Kimmy Hise

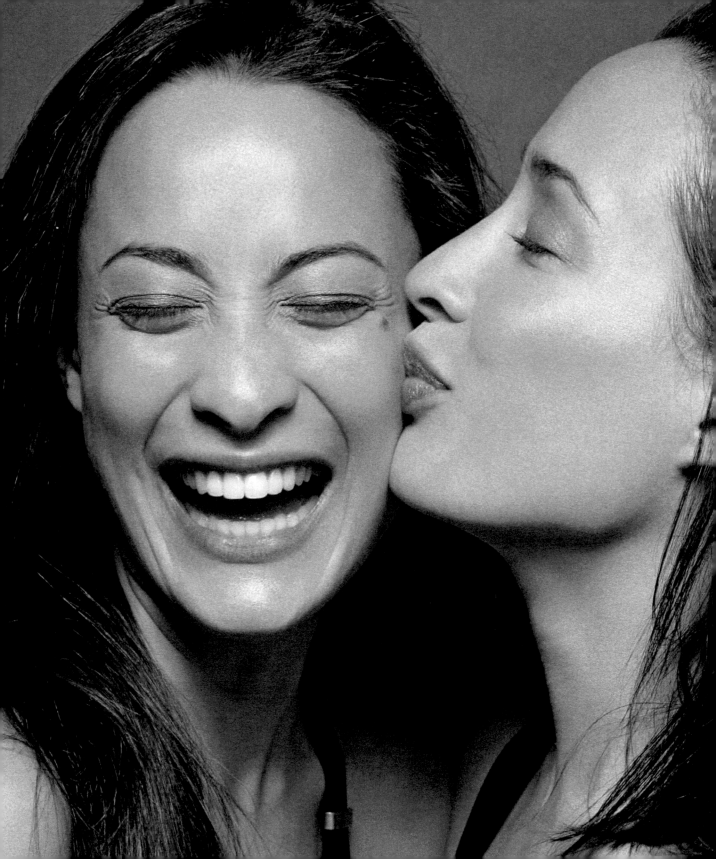

"You had me at 'hello.'"
—Renée Zellweger as Dorothy, *Jerry Maguire* (1996)

Have you ever looked across a room and someone just catches your eye? You are drawn to them, yet you can't quite put your finger on what it was that captured your attention.

Think back to someone you clicked with instantly. What was it about them? Maybe it was the way they laughed, which perhaps even made you laugh, for no reason at all. Maybe it was their smile, which warmed your heart. Or maybe it was just the way they moved through the room, which instantly put you at ease. All of us, at some point or another, have encountered this person. You may have heard someone say, "There's a certain *je ne sais quoi* about her that I find irresistible!" What is that intangible quality—literally the "I know not what"—that makes someone stand out from the rest?

The answer is: It is a natural, external chemistry. Now imagine yourself attracting that reaction whenever you enter a room. Having trouble picturing it? That's because you can't make it happen. You have to keep stirring up the chemistry within, and eventually your natural sparkle will combust.

That's what we are working on, together, in this book. Keep going. You're doing great!

There are so many variables as to why a natural attraction occurs. And because it's not forced and is generally a largely emotional response, it is a result of complete, unselfconscious honesty. It's about trusting your instincts and taking yourself by surprise. It's about forgetting what you think *should* happen and just letting things happen.

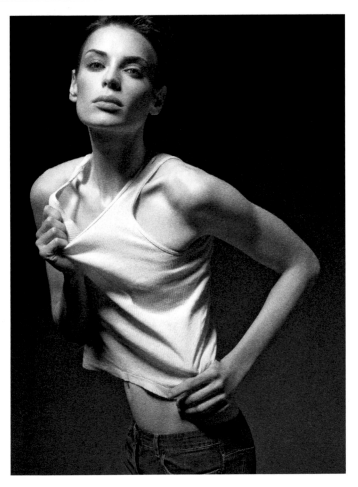

"I think spontaneity is crucial to being beautiful. When you are young, you don't care, and you go for it. When you are older, you start to think of responsibility, schedules, and so forth. Spontaneity is what keeps you young!"
—Yoanna House

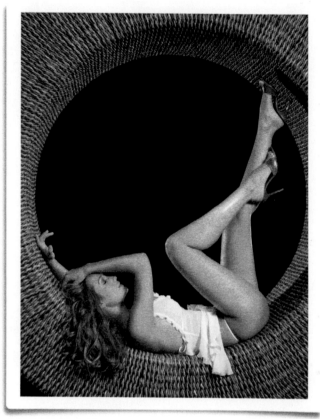

Supermodel Manon von Gerkan

"IT"

"'It' is that quality possessed by some which draws all others with its magnetic force.
With 'it' you win all men if you are a woman—all women if you are a man.
'It' can be a quality of the mind as well as a physical attraction."
—Novelist and screenwriter Elinor Glyn, describing actress Clara Bow in the Hollywood silent film *It* (1927)

CHECK OUT THESE FEMALE PARAGONS OF
THE "IT" FACTOR THROUGH THE LAST CENTURY

- CLARA BOW in *It* (1927)
- JEAN HARLOW in *Bombshell* (1933)
- JOSEPHINE BAKER in *Princesse Tam Tam* (1935)
- RITA HAYWORTH in *Gilda* (1946)
- MARILYN MONROE in *Gentlemen Prefer Blondes* (1953)
- AUDREY HEPBURN in *Breakfast at Tiffany's* (1961)

- DIANA ROSS in *Mahogany* (1975)
- DIANE KEATON in *Annie Hall* (1977)
- PHOEBE CATES in *Fast Times at Ridgemont High* (1982)
- JULIA ROBERTS in *Pretty Woman* (1990)
- PARKER POSEY in *Party Girl* (1995)
- ANNE HATHAWAY in *The Devil Wears Prada* (2006)

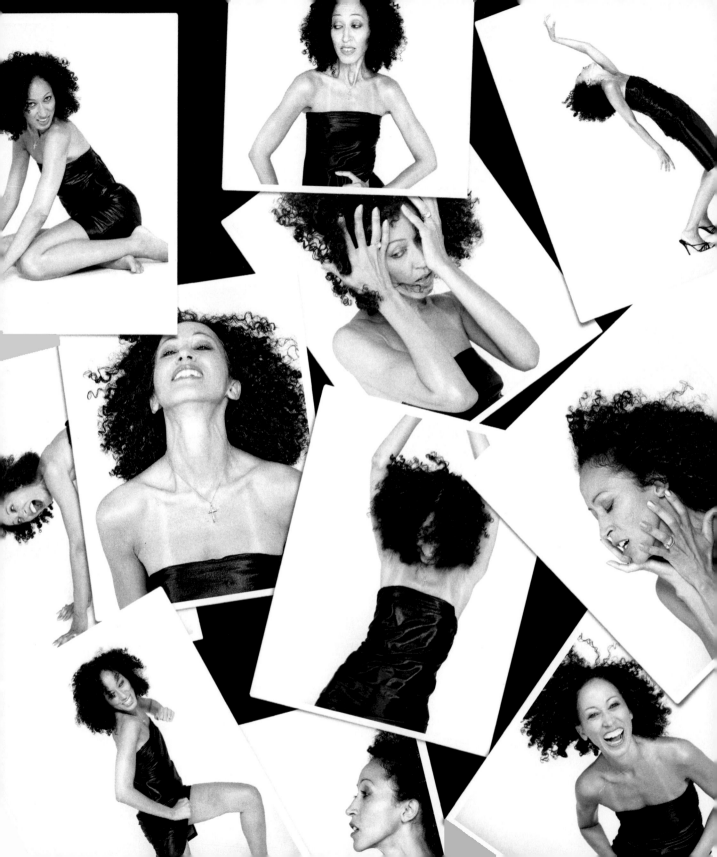

THAT'S THE SHOT

As a photographer, the magic moment when someone's natural chemistry shines through is the moment I must capture on film. That's the shot every client is looking for and the one everyone, whether thumbing through a magazine, surfing the Internet, or passing by a billboard, stops to see. Something that lures you in and entices you, that leads you to want to know more, that makes you want to run out and buy the perfume being advertised or the dress being worn—simply because the model selling it is creating a spontaneous moment within you, making you act on curiosity, impulse, and joy.

Capturing that moment in a portrait as a "voyeur" sounds easier than it is. I've had years of practice and have developed techniques (and the occasional magic trick), so luckily I can usually find the chemistry on my radar and harness and record it. But I can't do it alone.

The model not only has to "bring it," but she also has to bring "it." When I feel that effortless magnetism glowing from a candid smile and catch a glimmer from expressive, confident eyes, my instincts rarely fail me. Real spontaneity: That's what it takes for that great picture to be born. There simply is no beauty to be captured without "it."

"Whenever I feel myself sinking into negativity, I just stay above the line, like a cat trying to stay out of the dark, deep waters; with that, a natural spontaneity follows. It's just too hard to swim against the flow. Following the light of the positive is the way."

—Pat Cleveland

SPONTANEOUS SUPERSTAR

PAT CLEVELAND

If you've never heard of legendary model Pat Cleveland, let me take a moment to fill you in. Pat is considered by many to be the best runway model ever. Her style, spontaneity, and charisma has made her one of the most in-demand models since the seventies (she is still being booked constantly). She was one of the first internationally acclaimed supermodels of color; she was the muse to legendary fashion icon Halston; and she was fun (she was a regular at Studio 54 during its heyday). In fact, Josephine Baker once insisted that if a movie were ever made detailing her fabulous life, Pat Cleveland would have to play the part.

I've had the good fortune to shoot Pat, and now call her a friend. She made her mark with her high-energy, dramatic photos, and believe me when I tell you that was all Pat. When she first walked into my studio, she was like a ray of light. Genuinely interested in what everyone had to say, charming, with an almost childlike innocence. It's no wonder she was discovered at age fourteen (by a *Vogue* editor) on the subway.

Knowing Pat today leads me to believe that her glorious spirit is the reason designers and magazines alike fawned over her. She was a muse—not just to Halston, but to so many who worked with her—and an inspiration. Trumping any single physical attribute, this trait was the reason for her success. Although Pat's an obvious beauty, to be a muse you have to be able to start a fire in someone when you meet them. Pat does that innately, radiating a joy and respect that feels like a breath of fresh air whenever she walks into a room.

THE MUSES

In Greek mythology, poetry, and literature, the Muses are the goddesses or spirits who inspire the creation of literature and the arts and sciences with their graces. They are, as follows:

- CALLIOPE, muse of epic poetry
- CLIO, muse of history
- ERATO, muse of lyric poetry
- EUTERPE, muse of music
- MELPOMENE, muse of tragedy
- POLYHYMNIA, muse of choral poetry
- TERPSICHORE, muse of dance
- THALIA, muse of comedy
- URANIA, muse of astronomy

And here are some real-life muses and the artists they inspired:

- FERNANDE OLIVIER, muse to Pablo Picasso
- AUDREY HEPBURN, muse to Hubert de Givenchy
- DOVIMA, muse to Richard Avedon
- YOKO ONO, muse to John Lennon
- SUZANNE FARRELL, muse to George Balanchine
- GALA, muse to Salvador Dalí
- LEE MILLER, muse to Man Ray

THREE WAYS TO START BECOMING YOUR OWN "IT" GIRL

1. BE YOURSELF, AND TAKE ME WITH YOU

I love to tell a subject, "Pretend I don't have a camera. Just be your lovely self." Certainly easier said than done. Some girls freeze up when that mysterious lens starts staring at them (others are able to completely forget about the camera and relax). If you've seen me helm a photo shoot on television, you know I am not quiet behind the lens. I usually chat with a girl through the whole shoot, trying to create natural conversation and a pleasant rapport. Sometimes a girl will clench her teeth and try to answer me, like a ventriloquist trying not to move her mouth. Forget about it—that's only going to look awkward. Keep this in mind later, when you do your photo challenges: Talk back to the camera! Smile! Laugh! Don't worry about looking perfect. Just be you, and when you edit the pictures, you'll find the right click of the shutter.

You are absolutely right in thinking that a shot of you midsentence won't be your most flattering. How many times have our friends taken a wretched candid shot of us midlaugh, midbite, or midblink, and then posted it on Facebook, totally embarrassing us? But trust me, I am here to up your Beauty Equation, not make you look unattractive or foolish. Because I know—and I want you to know, and take this with you into your photo assignments and your life—that the second before you crack a smile or right after you stop giggling can be a moment of rare beauty, and . . . *snap!* Whoever was looking at you right then just got a million-dollar shot of you at your best.

If you need to, you can carry "me" out into the world. Imagine I am there, protecting you, wanting to see the most beautiful you. But if the image of me and my camera frightens you, then picture someone else, someone who loves you unconditionally. You can do no wrong in their eyes. That's how you need to imagine the world seeing you. You need the freedom to be "wrong," because that's the key to spontaneity. To be truly free, you have to allow yourself to feel potentially silly or awkward, while paradoxically trusting that you won't.

Perfection is a myth. If you try to get all your ducks in a row and wait until you are 100 percent sure everything is right before you make a move, you'll never make a move. If you don't enjoy things that happen to you spontaneously, it is very difficult to look natural and have any real chemistry with anyone in any situation, let alone everyone in every situation. It's all about keeping it real. No faking in front of the camera; it can tell every time. No faking in real life; it will backfire every time.

Consider this quote from e. e. cummings, arguably one of the most spontaneous poets ever to grace the planet (even the way he writes his name, in all lowercase, expresses spontaneity): "We do not believe in ourselves until someone reveals that deep inside us something is valuable, worth listening to, worthy of our trust, sacred to our touch. Once we believe in ourselves we can risk curiosity, wonder, spontaneous delight, or any experience that reveals the human spirit."

So guess what? It's time to believe. Feel worthy! Risk curiosity! Reveal your human spirit!

2. DO THE MATH, AGAIN

I can't stress this enough: All the other elements of the Beauty Equation figure into the subset of the formula for spontaneity. If you fear being naturally spontaneous, you have to go back and rethink the things I've talked about in the first three chapters. You have to have allure, always knowing you are presenting yourself in the best light, so that you can let your guard down and be the one and only you. You have to have the confidence to trust yourself, so you can take yourself by surprise. You must be compassionate, not just to others but also to yourself, so you can give yourself a break. Altogether, this adds up to a fabulous and smashing you. Total dynamite.

It doesn't matter if you are fast or slow when it comes to spontaneity. Take your time; talk back to life. It's about your curiosity. It's about taking a chance. It's about thinking outside the box. It's about enjoying your life and your work, and having fun.

Most of the growing you will do in life will come from taking a leap in the dark. You don't think about it; you just do it. Never done it before? You are now! Think about when you laugh—you don't plan it, do you? You can't. Something is just plain frickin' hilarious, and you have a spontaneous outburst called laughter. Where did it come from? Who planned it? Who cares? It's uninhibited and filled with surprises. *You* are uninhibited and filled with surprises.

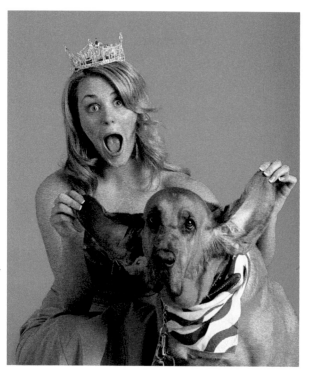

Lauren Nelson, Miss America 2007, caught in a quirky moment

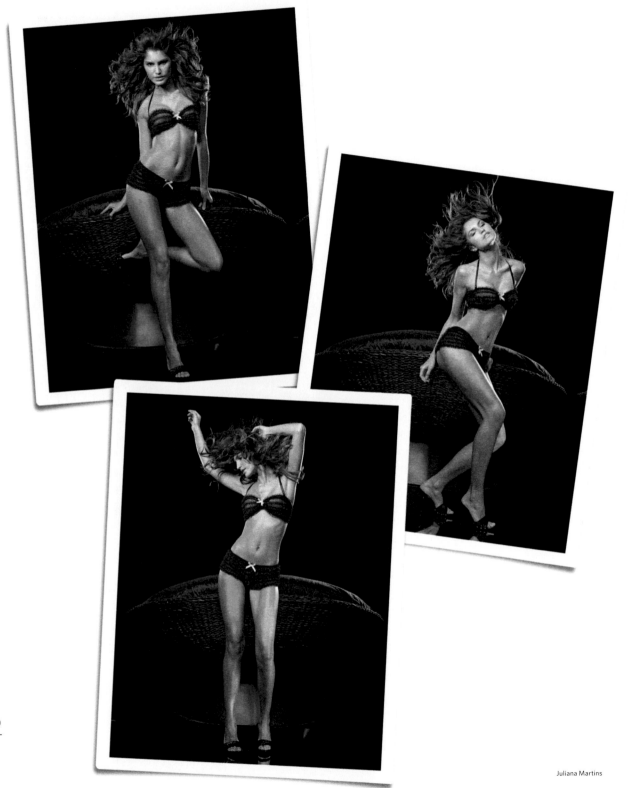

Juliana Martins

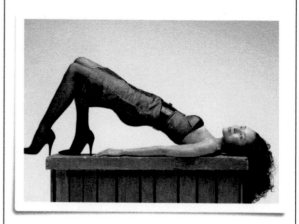

3. BE SPONTANEOUS, AND NOW DO IT AGAIN!

As we've discussed earlier, you can improve through practice. Yes, you can practice spontaneity. Remember, you don't lose for trying and you only get better the more times you walk down the proverbial runway.

DANCER IN THE DARK

Shut yourself in your room and put on your music player with headphones. Better yet, wait until you have the place to yourself. Then go to the biggest room in the house and turn out the lights. Now, put on your empowering theme song and crank it. Don't think. Let loose. Let your body do the talking. Interpret the music through your movement in a completely instinctual way. Remember, there is no one there judging you. It's just you dancing in the dark and hopefully having a blast. When the song is done, reflect on your mood. Were you able to let go? Did you feel the moves just came out of you from within? Put the song on again or create a playlist of groovy beats. Keep dancing and free your mind from analyzing the music. You're living off the wall!

PROFILE IN SPONTANEITY

APRIL WILKNER

April is at ease in most any situation off camera and can always bring it behind the lens. She is spontaneous. She can walk in and find out she is going to be suspended over a deep, cavernous hole by a single cable or that she will be posing in a flowing gown while completely submerged in water, and she'll seize the moment. She does things for the first time like she's done them dozens of times before and regularly delivers a beautiful picture. She can bring together all the things she might be learning in the moment by not thinking too hard about them and by letting her subconscious do the work. She can let her guard down and isn't afraid to take a chance. She's demonstrated she is a talented actress and dancer. But when it comes to posing with snakes in a photo shoot? Well, nobody can do it all, but those who try come out on top.

As a result of being so natural on camera, April was offered a job as host for the live broadcast of *CoverGirl's Talk Model*—the *Top Model Internet Talk Show*. You want to talk about spontaneity? Try doing a live show! In fact, really try it.

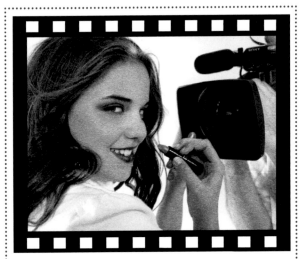

Carly Sheffield

Quick Video Challenge

As you work your way through your own Beauty Equation, you will come across "Quick Challenges" that encourage you to further explore the ten essential elements discussed in the book. Think of these challenges as surprise pop quizzes (but without the grades). You can choose to keep them private, or you can upload your experiences to your portfolio online under "Quickies." Have a go at it!

Invite a friend over, then set your music player to play some of your favorite tunes. Now act like you're doing an Internet radio show and give yourself thirty seconds of "airtime" to videotape yourself talking to an imaginary audience in between songs. It's harder than you think!

PARTY IT UP

Look at your engagement calendar. Look at your Facebook and your Twitter and your e-mail and your cell phone. See how many invitation requests you have pending, whether for a house party, school function, art opening, book signing, play, or a band. Now RSVP "yes" to all of them. If you've been invited to something, it's probably a pretty safe environment for you to go and be yourself.

When you go, you are not going to linger in the back and be a wallflower. You are going to say hello to everyone. Not just the friends you know, but the friends you don't know yet. Introduce yourself! See what you have in common. Be spontaneous. Be fun. Have fun.

If this is difficult or painful for you today, it's all the more important that you do it. Meeting new people in safe environments is a great way to develop your spontaneity. You never know what the other person is going to say, what you are going to have to talk about, or what the situation will call for. But you will learn and get better, and pretty soon, you'll be able to apply these skills to any circumstance.

NIGHT AT THE IMPROV

There are comedy clubs all over the world. Many of these clubs offer improvisational comedy classes or can lead you to a place that does. Improv puts you on the spot in front of others. If this sounds absolutely petrifying, don't worry—it is. The great thing in a class of beginners is that you are not alone. Everyone is scared to death. But with practice and through seeing others practice you can really begin to engage in a new level of spontaneity. If you've ever seen improv live or on television, you know how good the talented ones are at thinking on their feet, delivering a witty retort, or moving the situation forward.

If you don't have the inclination or funds to attend such a class, check out a book on the subject from the public library. There are many titles available. Gather a group of friends and practice the fundamentals. Just getting up and pulling a situation, emotion, or word out of the hat and running with it will get you going.

CHARADES

Another simple way to improve your ability to think on your feet is to get a group together and play charades. And don't be the one who sits back and guesses. Get up there and be the one to act it out! You know how to play charades, right? Someone has a secret phrase, movie title, book, TV show, or celebrity in mind. They have to get up in front of everyone and, without speaking, act out clues that help the others guess the secret. The more creative you are, the better the crowd can figure out your phrase. "Sounds like . . ."

THE NUMBER-ONE RULE OF IMPROV: What do you think the principal rule of improv is? What allows people to get up onstage together and create sketch comedy on the spot, with no script? It's the same rule that applies to spontaneous people in real life. It's so simple: Don't say "no." Don't say "I can't." Don't say "I won't."

In other words, don't stop the action. Keep it propelling forward. If you are at an interview and the potential boss asks, "Do you like hamburgers?" and you reply, "Ummm, no"—well, that's it, isn't it? End of story. But when you answer with a positive, even if you detest hamburgers and are a vegan, you keep the story going. You stay engaged. Answer with, "I'm a vegetarian and make the most awesome veggie burgers on the planet!" Be positive. Lead the situation into territory you are familiar with. If someone asks you if you like reality television, be honest, but don't stop the conversation. When you answer, "No, I hate that crap!" chances are, the conversation's over. That may be exactly how you feel, but try answering with, "The shows I do love are *CSI* and *Gossip Girl*!" Try it! As you will learn from the exercise "Night at the Improv," once someone says no, the show is over.

A FINAL WORD—UNNATURAL CHEMISTRY

On rare occasions, I've had the regrettable duty of having to let a model go or refusing to hire her because of her use of alcohol or other substances. Often, these girls feel that they are incapable of letting go of their inhibitions and being spontaneous, so they muster up some "liquid confidence" or "Dutch courage" in hopes of overcoming their insecurities and wowing everyone. Well, there's not much to say on this topic. Unfortunately, an intoxicated person is not a free spirit and is not likely to make rational decisions either. The false confidence you gain from substance abuse doesn't equal beauty. Just don't even go there.

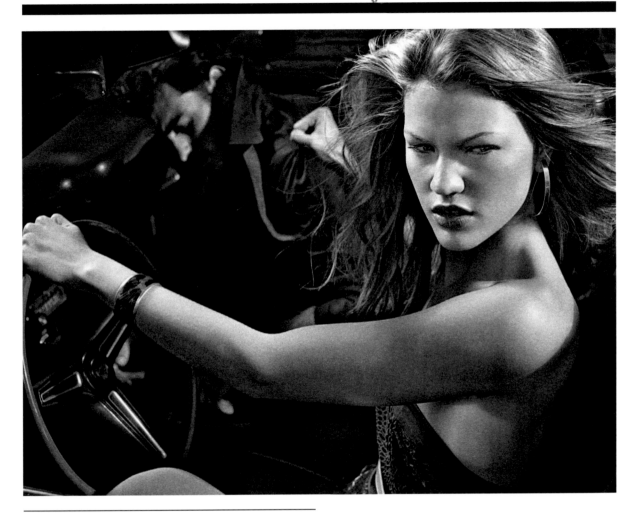

1. NATURAL FLOW

Have a look at these pictures I've taken over the next few pages. They suggest a story between the people involved in the action, don't you think? But there is no text—that's your job. Without any further guidance or requirements, look at the images, imagine the underlying plot that they suggest to you, and then go to your online or printed portfolio and give me a narrative about this picture. There is no right or wrong. Make it all up, but make it interesting and entertaining. Who is doing what to whom and why? Write!

Don't read any further until you've completed the writing challenge. The whole point is to get your spontaneous juices flowing. I'm sure once you started to create the story, you found your creativity and curiosity ready to go. If this was difficult for you, you must practice. Go pick up a random magazine or illustrated book in your house. Art books, photography books, or fashion magazines are all great. Open to a random page with a photo, and don't think twice. Write out a narrative. Keep doing this until you realize you can think on your feet and hit the ground running in any situation.

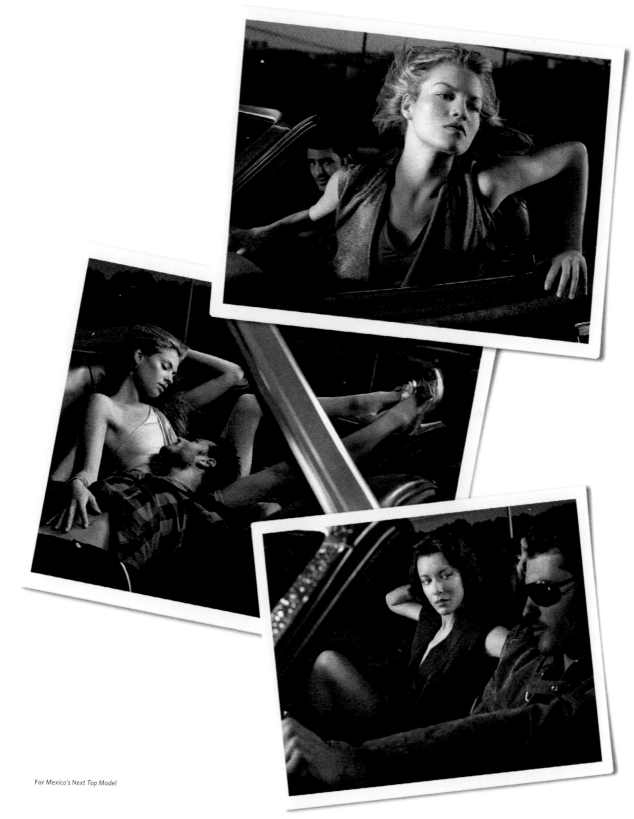

For *Mexico's Next Top Model*

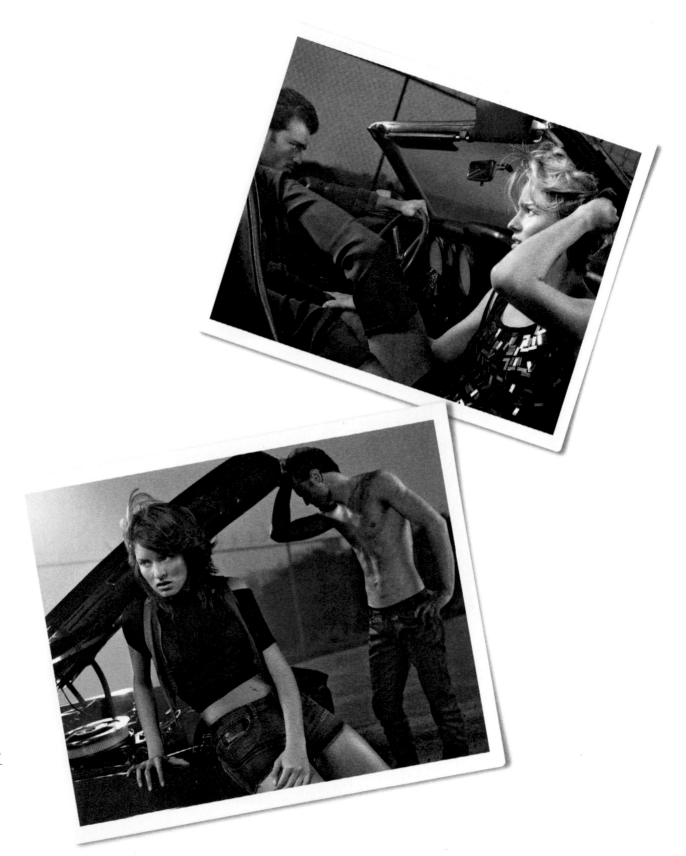

Let's go to the mall today! Nearly every shopping center has a photo booth, where you usually get three or four pictures for a few dollars. Once you insert your money, the booth automatically starts taking pictures in quick succession, allowing you just a moment in between to change your pose. Before you go to the mall, write the following emotions on little slips of paper:

Joy. Fear. Anger. Regret.
Surprise. Confidence. Love. Fury.
Confusion. Indifference.

OK, now blindly pick four of the slips and don't look at them. Slip them into your purse or your pocket. Only look at them once you are in the photo booth at the mall. Convey those emotions. Take the results and put them in your portfolio.

Set your camera on autotimer and just start telling a story. Don't look at the camera; look at an imaginary "me" beyond the camera and tell me what you had for breakfast, not neglecting a detail. Let the camera snap. Do it again, but this time, tell me about your favorite pet. *Snap!* Tell me a joke. *Snap!* Tell me a secret. *Snap!* After you've taken ten or so photos, review them. Some might be awkward or unflattering. *Delete!* But if you find one that reveals your candid beauty, add it to your portfolio. If you aren't happy with any of them, it's back to the drawing board. As an option, take ten more sitting in profile to the camera, with a mirror placed in front of you so you can see yourself in action.

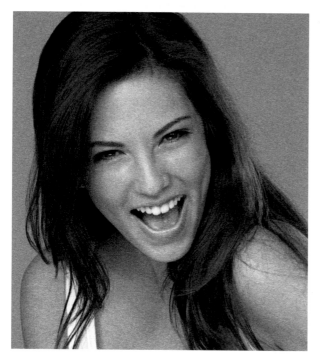

WE all have our own formula, or chemistry, a set of elements specific to us that determines who we are. Not just scientifically, but emotionally. Sure, we all have specific genes that make us unique, but it's also about how you wear those jeans that sends a particular message. Do you wiggle your hips? Do you cross your legs? Do you stomp around? Or do you skip? Everything we do and say, from the way we talk to the way we move and dress to the way we act, all adds up to how people perceive us. Childlike innocence is just as beautiful as educated smarts when offered up with charm and dignity. The trick is to try to be the best you and let your natural chemistry show.

Rachel Oyama, twenty-four, aspiring actress, capturing spontaneity

87

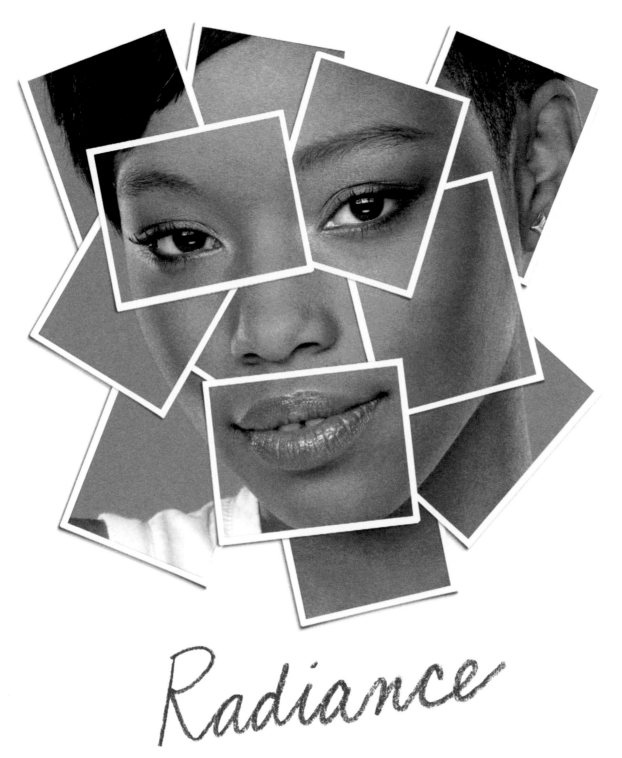

Radiance

TO ENHANCE THE BRILLIANCE OF YOUR INNER GLOW

Skin-Deep: *the teach*

MIRROR, MIRROR, ON THE WALL

What do you see when you look in the mirror? Do you study your face, looking for the slightest imperfection? Are you constantly on the lookout for an uninvited hair or the first sign of a blemish? Have you ever stared at your face for so long you can no longer judge what you are even looking at? Well, stop all of that nonsense right now! The mirror can be your friend, but it is not a gateway to your magnificence. It is merely a mathematical tool in the Beauty Equation: It functions like a plus or a minus sign, depending upon your level of self-esteem when you gaze into it. In other words, you can't count on it until you can control the roller coaster of self-perception affecting what you see. And who can really ever do that? It's a healthy part of human nature to question ourselves. Just not too much. Or too little. And that is the basic rule of thumb for this chapter, because we are talking about outer presentation—the way in which your skin, hair, and clothes tell your inner story.

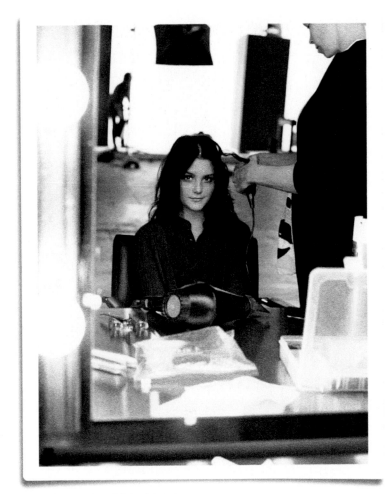

Madeline Finnegan getting ready for her photo shoot

Sometimes I feel a bit like a mirror when I'm behind my camera. When I'm creating a *beauty shot*, a term we use in the fashion industry to describe a photo that is totally focused on a model's face, I use what is known as a long lens. It allows me to be far enough away that I'm not right in your face, but allows me to zoom in to the point where it's almost like I'm looking through a microscope. This process gives me an all-access pass to the human face. I can see every pore and crease. I can stare with an eaglelike focus into the eyes and watch as the pupils dilate and contract, allowing me into the thoughts that come and go from the mind's eye. My long lens allows me to visualize your face like a topographical map and reveals to me the ups and downs of your life, as well as the peaks and valleys of your skin.

But as a mirror, I'm not like the magic mirror in *Snow White*, which would taunt the Evil Queen whenever she asked who was the "fairest of them all," by telling her Snow White was far more beautiful. I'm not scrutinizing you for your flaws. I watch your lips, waiting for that quiver or lick to reveal what you might be suggesting. I look for the flattering lines around your eyes or mouth, to see if a smile or jeer might be forthcoming. I might try to make you laugh, or praise you, or surprise you. I am on a quest for radiance and I won't quit until I tap into yours.

So guess what? It's time to look in the mirror. To see what the world sees. It's time to learn how to present yourself in order to radiate your *true self*.

ANTM contestant Anya Rozova

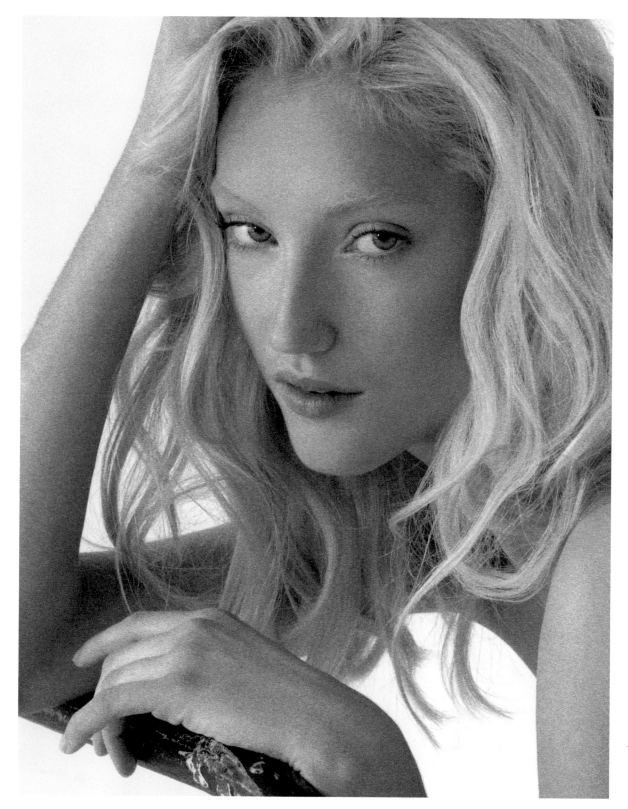

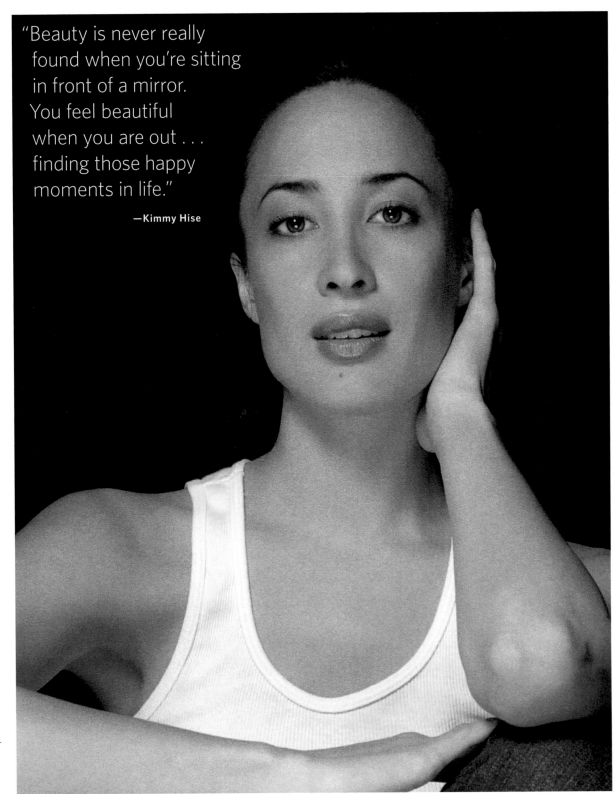

"Beauty is never really
found when you're sitting
in front of a mirror.
You feel beautiful
when you are out . . .
finding those happy
moments in life."

—Kimmy Hise

DANGEROUS BEAUTY AHEAD!

The oft-repeated phrase "Beauty is only *skin-deep*" originated in the seventeenth century, as a way of saying that physical beauty is superficial and true beauty comes from within. Of course, I know from experience, and you do too, that you can be tricked by someone's facade. But deep down we all know that you should judge a person by their actions and character rather than by the way they look.

Just as everyone is innocent until proven guilty, everyone is beautiful until proven ugly. And ugliness usually has to do with having an underlying mean spirit, which gets reflected in the way you present yourself.

Have you ever been honked at and flipped off by a "beautiful" person barreling down the freeway (while talking on a cell phone) or yelled at simply because you choose to drive safely and responsibly? That's ugly. (And I should know—it's happened to me. Someone filled with road rage actually screamed, "White trash!" at me from their car!)

Anyway, the point is that you send a message about who you are by how you behave as well as how you look. Ask yourself, what is the image I am trying to project? Every decision you make, from the way you vent your frustration on the road to the makeup you put on and the designer you wear has an association with your inner character.

Developing the inner self is up to each individual and takes the kind of hard work we have been doing together in this book. Changing your outer appearance to reflect the most beautiful you may seem like a simple matter of style, but it also requires understanding yourself within, so you know who to project!

Ready to start your makeover?

If beauty is skin-deep, let's start there!

THE FEMME FATALE

Femme fatale is a French term that literally means "disastrous woman." An incredibly radiant and alluring woman who is an archetype in literature and film, her beauty is truly only skin-deep. She uses her feminine wiles to fool innocent victims, wreaking havoc wherever she goes. Don't be seduced by this she-wolf in sheep's clothing. She has a black heart and will get you every time. (And she always gets her comeuppance in the end.)

FIVE MODERN FEMME FATALES

1. DIANE KRUGER in *Inglourious Basterds* (2009)

2. SARAH MICHELLE GELLER in *Cruel Intentions* (1999)

3. NICOLE KIDMAN in *To Die For* (1995)

4. SHARON STONE in *Basic Instinct* (1992)

5. KATHLEEN TURNER in *Body Heat* (1981)

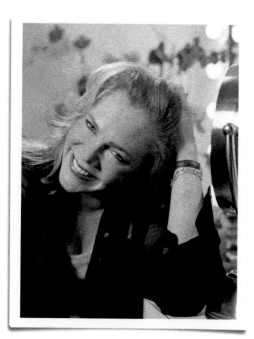

Kathleen Turner, actress

THE SKINNY ON SKIN

So we know that you can change your "skin-deep" persona through your words and actions. That being said, taking extremely good care of your precious skin is a gift you can give yourself that will keep giving back for years to come. This also applies to your hair, your body, and even your wardrobe. Bring these values to your Beauty Equation and you'll find your solution adding up.

"People are like stained-glass windows: They sparkle and shine when the sun is out, but when the darkness sets in, their true beauty is revealed only if there is a light from within."

—Elisabeth Kübler-Ross, psychiatrist and writer

Tyra once said, "I love the confidence that makeup gives me." In the right proportions, makeup can enhance your natural features and, combined with your innate beauty bring about radiance—our goal here. Too much makeup, on the other hand, can hide your beauty, or even produce a comic effect. I've had several incredibly striking female models reveal to me that, when they've overdone their makeup before going out, they've been told, "You look so great, no one would even know you're a man!" There's a time and a place for everything. Unless you're a drag queen, the time for overdoing it is called Halloween, and that only comes once a year. Makeup is a great tool and can be used to take you from sophisticated and glamorous to hippie chic to conservative and classic. Just don't go overboard in your desire to look dramatic. You can do that just with the sparkle in your eyes.

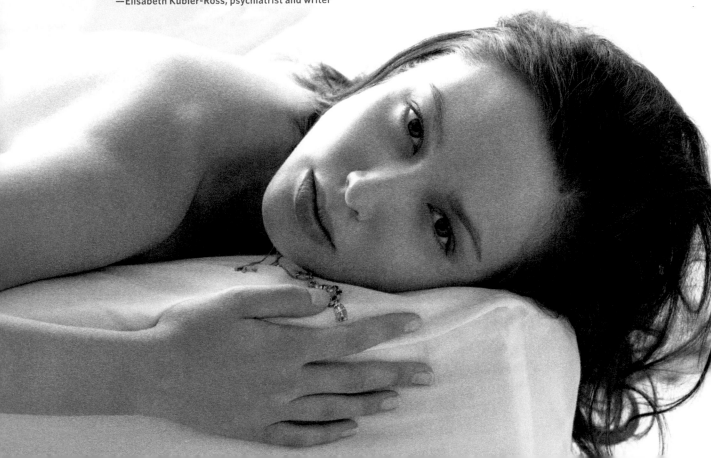

MAKEUP DOs AND DON'Ts

DO

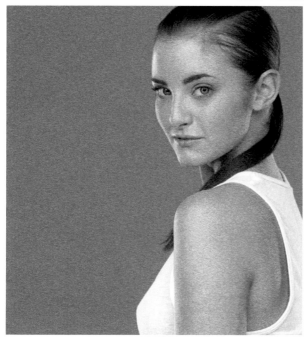

Nicole Ray Muller

LOVE YOUR SKIN

Your skin is the largest and most visible of your organs. It is a living, breathing thing, just like your heart. Treat it well and give it respect, and it will gain you props in return. Never put on makeup without first being sure your skin is freshly washed and moisturized. By the same token, at the end of the night, take the time to remove your makeup and leave your skin as fresh and clean as before you put it on. You'll be saving your skin (and your pillowcase) for a long and prosperous run.

TRICKS OF THE TRADE: Drink plenty of water. This will help your skin glow and ward off dryness. Exfoliate once a week, and treat your face to a steam bath. Try putting some essential oil in the water for a relaxing facial.

Kaiulani Swan

SEE THE LIGHT

If you want people to see you in a perfect light, give yourself the perfect light when you put your face on. Make sure there is a bright, even light by your mirror (don't use your rearview mirror or a compact). Make sure you don't leave anything to chance. Do your makeup before you go out and—equally important—check it in the same type of light you are going out in.

When I was young, my mother had a portable makeup mirror that plugged in and simulated different lighting settings: day or evening, home or office. Although these fascinating devices are no longer in vogue today, you can take a lesson from my mother, who always viewed herself in the light she was going to be seen in and did her makeup accordingly. Think about where you are going and try to imitate that light somewhere at home before you go out—location, location, location! Heading to a dark nightclub for some jazz? Turn off all the lights in your room except for a side lamp and see if you have done your eyes too lightly. Invited to a daytime premiere on the red carpet, with bright lights and flashbulbs? Take a hand mirror out into the backyard and stand in the sunniest spot you can find to make sure your foundation looks 100 percent even. Then don't forget to check yourself out under the dining room chandelier to make sure you'll look great in the amber glow of the lobby lights too.

TRICKS OF THE TRADE: Study your face in different lighting using the shadows and highlights that are cast on your visage to learn how light can affect the way your features look. Think about how you can use different products to mimic these effects. Don't underestimate the power of a good bronzer here—it is a great way to add subtle contours to your face.

REMEMBER, LESS IS MORE

I promise you: The less makeup you wear, the more you shine through. Experiment and see what products bring out your best features. It is not a requirement that you use foundation, eyeliner, mascara, eye shadow, rouge, lipstick, lip gloss, bronzer, and concealer just because they exist. Find the bare bones of makeup you need to impress according to your own unique equation.

If longer eyelashes is all it takes for you to dazzle, so be it. (Bear in mind that sometimes an eyelash curler is more effective than a coat of mascara—and sometimes fake eyelashes make your peepers pop). Figure out what works, but as a rule of thumb, keep it minimal, classic, and classy, and it's hard to go wrong.

TRICKS OF THE TRADE: Makeup artists live by the rule that you should have either a strong lip or a strong eye—never both. Unless you are doing an edgy fashion shoot, take it from the pros and stick to this rule as well.

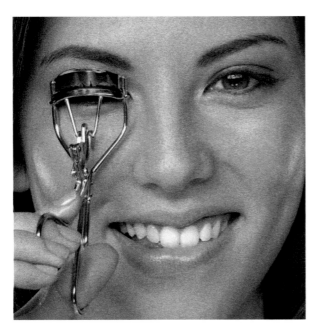

Rachel Oyama

BLUR THE LINES

Blend your makeup! You don't want to see where one color ends and another one starts. And you really don't want any hard lines, especially when it comes to lip liner. This is the drag queen's staple and the natural beauty's downfall. Subtlety is an art. You don't want people to see your makeup; you want them to see you.

TRICKS OF THE TRADE: When applying your foundation, try using a sponge that has been moistened in water first. This will help dilute the product and give you a sheer and even application.

When you're done with your makeup, take a moment to brush over your face lightly with a big, fluffy brush, using a circular motion to make sure everything is blended. Don't forget your neck and your hairline.

PROTECT THE INNOCENT

Don't subject your clothes to your makeup regimen. Apply your makeup in a bathrobe or cover your outfit with a towel. Your clothes won't wear it well.

And while we're talking about the innocent, do all you can to protect the guiltless creatures that lose their lives or are subjected to suffering in the name of research and development of cosmetics. It has never been easier to find cruelty-free makeup and beauty products. Organizations like People for the Ethical Treatment of Animals (PETA) have online databases that allow you to look up companies and brands that produce beauty products without harming animals. Don't support testing lipstick and eye shadow on rabbits. They are beautiful just the way they are!

TRICKS OF THE TRADE: Having your upper chest exposed while you apply your makeup is the best way to ensure that the skin tone of your face matches the rest of your body.

PRACTICE, PRACTICE, PRACTICE

You want to put your best face forward. Practice at home when you have nowhere to go and there's no pressure to perfect your makeup technique. Try new things and see what works for you. Get feedback from people you trust. Remember, there is no set rule for how makeup works. You must find the solution and then remember the equation. Makeup application is 10 percent skill and 90 percent practice.

TRICKS OF THE TRADE: A great way to try out a new makeup technique or look is to practice on someone else. So become a makeup artist for a day—it is an eye-opening experience to face your subject and approach a whole new set of features. And if they return the favor, you may even end up with a few new tricks up your sleeve.

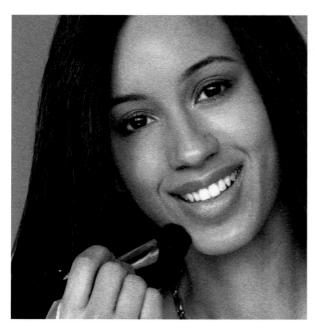

Roselyn Azcona

DON'T

DON'T REFLECT TOO MUCH

Avoid using too much in the way of shimmery high-lights or makeup that refracts light. In the wrong light, it looks unnatural and awkward, and in photos it can catch the light in an unflattering manner.

TRICKS OF THE TRADE: You want to have contours on your face, not a big, shiny mess. Light pops features out, and dark pushes features in. To play with the light, makeup artists use shimmer along the bridge of the nose, dotted on the inner corner of the eye, and dusted on the apples of the cheeks.

DON'T COVER UP

Trying to conceal real skin problems does more harm than good. When you have acne or a similar condition, covering it with heavy makeup is only going to make your skin condition worse. The camera sees all, and so will everyone else! Relax. Take the time to remedy your skin ailment before you use any makeup. Short-term results are just that, short-term. Think about the long run and you'll end up a winner.

TRICKS OF THE TRADE: Remember the trick above about light and dark shades? If you have a minor blem-ish (and not a bad case of acne, as discussed above), if you cover it with a shade that is too light, it will stand out even more. Try using a dab of foundation match-ing your skin tone, dusted lightly with powder. If the blemish is on your cheek, you can mix a little cream blush with the foundation so your coverage will not stand out.

Chamomile is a natural anti-inflammatory and can work wonders for a pesky blemish. Use it in a tea bag as a warm compress, being careful not to burn your skin. This also works great for tired, puffy eyes, only this time, chill your moistened tea bag.

DON'T CLASH

Your skin tone is unique. You want to play up this sin-gular quality that only you have. Don't draw attention away from your tone by using colors that have noth-ing to do with you. They will stand out and detract from your overall package. Try to find the shades that match and complement your colors. And when you find a foundation that matches your skin, stock up on it (just check the expiration date and store it well). You know how companies love to discontinue the one thing you love!

TRICKS OF THE TRADE: Your skin tone darkens and lightens with the seasons. You should have two shades of foundation to play with so that you always have the perfect match. If you want to take it to the next level, try mixing the two shades on your hand to create your own custom blend.

DON'T BE A VICTIM

Beware of the friendly person behind the mall makeup counter. They are there for one reason: to sell as much as possible. You can have fun with them and listen to what they have to say; some are professional makeup artists with real insight to impart. But some are sea-sonal hires who work on commission and will tell you anything it takes to get you to walk away with way more makeup than you need.

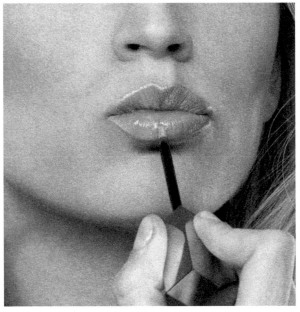

Shannon Rusbuldt

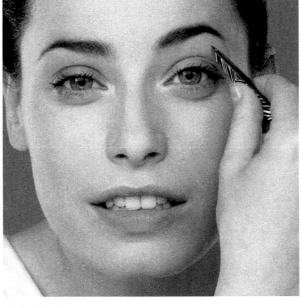

Yuilya Malamud

TRICKS OF THE TRADE: It's often helpful to bring a friend with you to the makeup counter for a second opinion. Feel free to step outside the store and check out your new look in daylight. You do not need to duplicate the whole look, either. Just pick and choose what works best for you. If you like what you're seeing, try to watch how the makeup artist applies your makeup in a mirror, and take mental notes.

DON'T BE LOWBROW

Don't overtweeze your eyebrows. Full brows have been in since the seventies and Brooke Shields. Getting carried away in any department is a surefire recipe for disaster, but this one can be hard to reverse. Follow the natural contour of your face when shaping. If you pluck too much, you will have that permanent look of surprise—and so will everybody else.

TRICKS OF THE TRADE: When it comes to plucking your eyebrows, follow these rules of thumb: Invest in good tweezers, and never pluck from the top of your brow—only along the bottom. Before you begin, brush your brows in an upward motion so that you can see what you're doing. A toothbrush works well. You want your brow to start at the inner corner and end at the outer corner of your eye, arching gently above your

iris. Pluck one hair at a time and step back to look at the whole picture frequently to avoid overplucking and to keep your brows even. Take it slow! You can always go back and tweeze more, but you can't undo what you've done.

DON'T FOOL YOURSELF

Don't try to make yourself over into someone you're not. Just because a makeup trend is hot or a certain technique looks great on someone in a magazine, that doesn't mean it's necessarily going to look great on you. It might, so try it. But if it doesn't work, don't force the issue. Look for what looks great on you.

TRICKS OF THE TRADE: Once again, you be the makeup artist. Try new things on someone else and then have them try new things on you. You'll have fun and see firsthand how what works for one might not work for all.

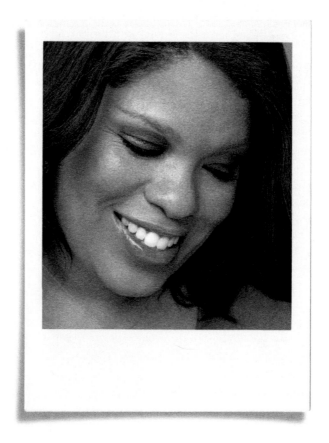

TOP TIPS FROM AN EXPERT

ANDREA DAWN CLARK

As beauty director of *Woman's World* magazine,
Andrea Dawn Clark is always writing beauty tips. Here are some of her favorites:

- Pick one feature to emphasize—your lips or your eyes and play up one while you downplay the other.
- Embrace your hair's natural texture. Have curly hair? If it's hot and humid outside, you're wasting your time blowing it out straight. When your curls are sopping wet, run some curl cream through them, and let the curls dry—beautifully defined—while you're out in the sun. Have straight hair? If it can't hold a curl skip the hot rollers and curling irons. Instead, get a cut that shows off your hair's natural sleekness.
- Realize that God gave you the features you have for a reason—mess with them and you might ruin his masterpiece.
- Never go to bed with your makeup on.
- Wear sunscreen and drink lots of water.
- Get some sleep!

MORE ON SKIN: A WRINKLE IN TIME

Your skin reflects a lot about you. For instance, if I met you in person and took your photo, I bet I could tell if you were a laugher or a frowner. Like your eyes, your face is a mirror. And whether you are radiating goodwill or malevolence will determine how your mirror will crack. I'm talking about wrinkles.

Look, wrinkles are a fact of life. But as much as I personally love them (because they show who you are and where you have been), I do everything I can to slow their arrival, and you should too. I'd rather all our skin stay as youthful as possible for as long as possible.

TO WRINKLE OR NOT TO WRINKLE

REMEMBER, THE SUN IS NOT YOUR FRIEND

Although it may feel good, soaking in the sun is the single most damaging thing you can do to your skin. Especially with the ozone layer quickly dissipating, the harmful ultraviolet rays from the sun can accelerate the aging process. Think about a raisin. Once a smooth, round grape, after sitting in the sun it becomes a dried-up, shriveled, and wrinkly little morsel.

The solution is actually rather simple. If you are going to be out in the sun, wear a hat with a broad brim and sunglasses. Stay in the shade as much as possible. It's a good daily practice to apply sunscreen first thing in the morning, since you're likely to be face-to-face with the fire in the sky at some point during your day.

DON'T STRESS OUT

I know—easier said than done. But you actually have a lot more control than you think over your stress, and constant stress can take its toll on your face. Make sure to treat yourself right. Take time out to meditate, treat yourself to a hot bath, and make sure you don't carry the day's tension to bed with you. Another great stress reliever is exercise. Doing thirty minutes of aerobic exercise a day will help take your mind off your worries, help you sleep, and do wonders for your skin. It doesn't have to be anything strenuous or require a trip to the gym. A brisk walk or bike ride will do the trick.

ALWAYS CARRY A SMILE WITH YOU

You are a happy person. Always remember that, and let the world know it with your smile. I guarantee you that when you put on a happy face, people see the smile and not the wrinkles. It's the easiest and most economical face-lift on the market.

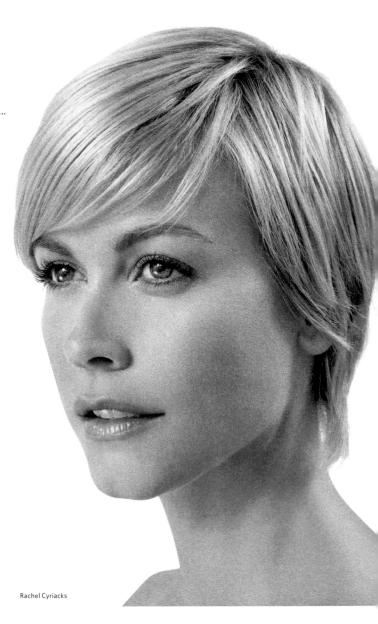

Rachel Cyriacks

> "It's a good thing that beauty is only skin-deep or I'd be rotten to the core."
>
> —Plastic-surgery-addicted comedienne Phyllis Diller

DON'T MASH YOUR FACE

My mother always used to tell us to be careful about "pulling faces," threatening that the "wind might change," and then that ugly look could get stuck there forever. What she meant was that if you are constantly furrowing your brow or making funny faces, you will train the lines in your forehead to become more prominent, or turn the lines around your eyes into crow's-feet. Take a sheet of paper and crumple it up into a ball, then unfold it again. What happens? What was once a flat, clean sheet now has permanent creases. Your skin reacts to repetition and will begin to hold the creases you subject it to over and over.

For further safekeeping, send your skin to night school! Make a good night cream part of your regular skin-care regimen. You'll wake up knowing your skin has been deeply moisturized and you have done your part in reducing sags and wrinkles. Remember, an ounce of prevention is worth a pound of cure.

KNOW YOUR KNOWN ENEMIES

To avoid unnecessary wrinkling, steer clear of the following three known enemies:

SMOKING: It is a proven fact that smoking cigarettes is wretched for your health, yet many succumb to the addiction. Believe me, I've seen many models puffing away off camera. But the fact remains that smoking cuts off oxygen, which nourishes the skin. Also, the constant puckering of the mouth around a cigarette can result in premature lines around your lips. The choice is yours.

DRINKING: I'm not a prude and I'm not advocating prohibition! I'm just reminding you to drink responsibly if you do drink. Excessive drinking can leave you with a puffy face in the morning. By the time that swelling goes down, your skin has already been stretched, and the constant pulling and pushing of your face can leave you with new wrinkles.

YO-YO DIETING: Similar to the effects of alcohol, if you lose and gain weight continually over time, your skin will expand and contract, stretch and shrink, and leave behind the little devils we are trying to avoid. Once you've put in the hard work and discipline it takes to adhere to a diet, don't give up on it! It's hard to travel down the same road and hurdle the same obstacles twice. Be proud of your achievement and hold on to it!

THE WRINKLES OF DORIAN GRAY

> "The reason I will not exhibit this picture is that I am afraid that I have shown in it the secret of my own soul."
>
> —*The Picture of Dorian Gray*, Oscar Wilde

The Picture of Dorian Gray is a classic novel of gothic horror by Oscar Wilde. It tells the story of a physically beautiful man named Dorian Gray who has his portrait done at the height of his good looks. However, deep in his heart, Dorian is a monster. So much so that he sells his soul in hopes that his portrait will display his aging and sinful living while he remains forever attractive and unaffected. In the end, the portrait serves as a reminder to him of the effect each dastardly act has upon the soul, with each offense manifested as a defect of his form or as premature wrinkles and the sags of age.

Over the years, I have photographed many a pretty face. But more often than you would imagine, I am reminded of the story of Dorian Gray. Why? Because no matter what kind of knockout walks through the door for a photo shoot, as soon as my camera starts clicking and I start interacting with the supposedly drop-dead-gorgeous model, she can rapidly start to lose her looks. I can, in fact, be knocked dead with surprise by the end of a shoot because the "beauty" I started with is walking out the door an unattractive bore. Even though the photos will turn out fine and people looking at them in a magazine might exclaim, "Why, isn't she something!", no amount of skill (or Photoshopping) can prevent conceit and egotism from shining through. Like many women, my mother can always see through a false face, and she has often looked at one of my photographs and said, "This girl is easy on the eye, but all I see is sheer arrogance!"

If you spend your time plotting the downfall of others, thinking ill of people, or just being your run-of-the-mill, all-around megabitch, the lines on your face will reflect it. The visual illusions created by those cheekbones you thought of as perfectly placed will be shattered.

Have you ever met a girl who is not conventionally pretty or a guy who is "not your type" and found them appealing anyway? I am always intrigued when this happens to me. People often ask if I can predict which girls will be the final three standing when I meet them initially on the first episode of *ANTM*. Absolutely not! I know better and reserve my judgment. Of course, the obviously pretty girls make an immediate impression, but eventually they show their true colors and many of them turn out to be unfriendly or uninspiring. The seemingly ungainly contestants, on the other hand, might end up revealing their beauty in a way that only their personal stories will allow for. So remember, by being charming, courteous, and, of course, willing and able, you can, like a chameleon, actually alter the way you appear to others.

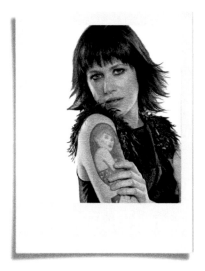

CASE IN POINT

SHANDI SULLIVAN

"After the series, I'd look in the mirror and feel really good inside. When I got on that show I didn't think much of myself. Yeah, I had a boyfriend, but so what? I thought, he thinks I'm cute, but no one else does."

When I first laid eyes on Shandi, I was speechless. Here was this shy girl with nerdy glasses, stringy hair, and schlumpy clothes who I basically sized up as what I will lovingly refer to her now as, a geek. The proverbial ugly duckling. But I didn't want to jump to conclusions based on first impressions. And it's a good thing I didn't!

Shandi, whose greatest achievement had been working as a clerk at Walgreens in Missouri, quickly blossomed. Why? Because as time went on, she learned how to reveal her radiance. Shandi naturally exhibits a charm, sincerity, and honesty that makes her beautiful. She has the determination and the ability to learn from her mistakes, to listen to advice, and to embrace change. She transformed herself from a small-town girl into a viable high-fashion model. Says Shandi, "Funny. It just took a haircut and contacts. But really, it was not just that." Shandi demonstrates that she has beauty where it really counts—inside—and a little hair, makeup, and fashion advice was all she needed to emerge as an undeniable beauty.

HAIR IT IS!

Your hairstyle, or lack thereof, also says a lot about you. People love a good makeover episode on TV. That's because we get to see how dramatically changing someone's hair changes the way we perceive them. Many women have a poor understanding of what makes them look beautiful when they sit down for a makeover. A good haircut and a change of color completely alters not only the viewers' perception of them, but also their perception of themselves.

(DOWNLOAD)

SONGS ABOUT... HAIR WITH RADIANCE

"Gimme a head with hair. Long beautiful hair. Shining, gleaming, streaming, flaxen, waxen!"

"Hair" —THE NEW BROADWAY CAST RECORDING

"My Hair Looks Fierce" —AMANDA LEPORE

"Hair" —ASHLEY TISDALE

"Hairspray Queen" —NIRVANA

"Platinum Blonde" —BLONDIE

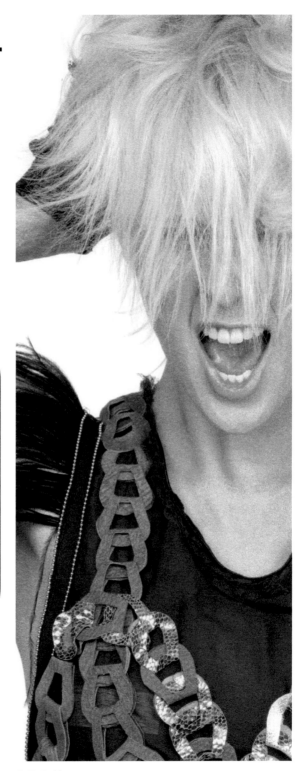

Caridee English

SIMPLE IS BETTER

I constantly advise models to pull their hair back in a ponytail or chignon (pronounced "sheen-yon"), which exposes your features and looks classic and elegant while accentuating your neck and your jawline.

SOMETIMES LESS IS, WELL, LESS

If you do nothing with your hair and let it fall where it may, you run the risk of looking like you've been dragged through a hedge backward. Your "I'm too cool to care" attitude might just come off as sloppy. Save bed head for pillow talk!

SOMETIMES MORE IS WAY TOO MUCH

When you use a ton of product, it suggests that you might have poorly treated or damaged hair. You may be thinking the "more the merrier," when quite frankly you could look like a tarred duck in an oil slick. Product is meant to control, shape, and contour. If you can see the product in your hair, it's too much.

YOU CAN LEAD YOUR HAIR TO WATER, BUT YOU HAVE TO MAKE IT DRINK

Healthy hair has a moisture content of 10 percent. When it drops below that level, it looks and feels dry. Good moisturizing conditioners have "humectants," which not only replace lost moisture but actually attract moisture and help the cortex of the hair retain it. Read the back label of your products. Price and design mean very little when it comes to making sure you are giving your hair what it needs. And sometimes the fancier brands put in additives to make the process of moisturizing feel more intense when the end result is no better. If it's hard to rinse off, it might be doing more harm than good.

WHEN IT COMES TO COLOR, "YOU'RE WORTH IT"

Coloring your hair can be a tricky business. Your natural hair has many, many colors in it. Good coloring by a hair-care professional is created using multiple streaks and layers, blending properly, and using after-treatments to remoisturize. A good dye job costs money but can give you spectacular results. If you are on a budget, home-color kits have made vast improvements in recent years and are a great alternative. You can achieve professional results at home, but take your time, and remember, you get what you pay for. Of course, the most economical solution of all is to learn to love your natural color!

YOUR NATURAL TEXTURE RULES

Go with your curly hair—it's gorgeous. Let your straight hair be your trademark—never, ever get a perm (it does terrible damage to your hair). Here are some ideas to toss around with your hairdresser: Straight hair loves a bob or a long, blunt cut. Curly hair loves layers. Coarse, thick hair is best kept medium to long, reducing bulk by varying lengths. Fine hair looks best all one length with layers around the face, and either very long or very short.

AN EXTRA RINSE CYCLE IS KEY

Make sure you rinse well; most shampoos are really too harsh for daily use. Think of your hair as the lettuce in a salad. You can clean it and wash it, but if you are too harsh with it, you'll bruise the leaves. And you definitely don't want any residual soap on it when you serve it up!

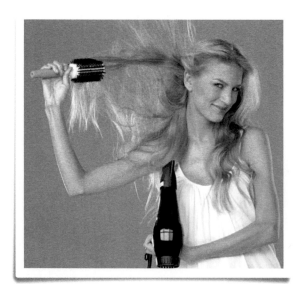

Shannon Rusbuldt

Quick Challenge

Jazz Up Your Hair

ANTM winner Jaslene Gonzalez demonstrates how to do a simple chignon.

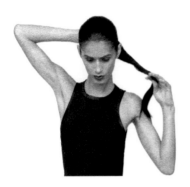 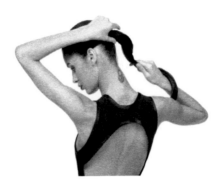 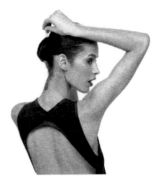

1. Completely dry your hair, using some styling product to give it some hold. Make sure you smooth out your hairline by bringing up the hairs at the nape of the neck.

2. Smooth your hair out and brush it into a ponytail, using a rubber band to hold it in place if needed.

3. Twist your ponytail onto itself to form your chignon, which is basically a bun on the back of your head. How small or large it is depends on your cut.

4. Once you have fully twisted your ponytail around to form the chignon, tuck the ends in and use large bobby pins the same color as your hair to secure it.

5. Finish with hair spray.

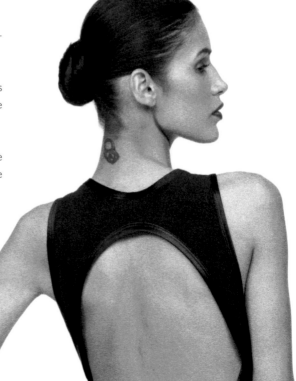

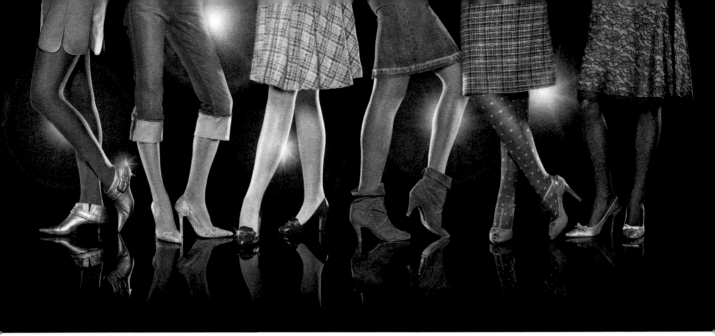

CLOTHES MAKE THE WOMAN

"Your dresses should be tight enough to show you're a woman and loose enough to show you're a lady."

—**Edith Head, costume designer**

Your clothing and fashion style speaks volumes about you. But unlike the process of enhancing the face and hair nature has given you, for which there are certain established guiding principles, your attire is completely your choice. There is no set of rules to follow when you are getting dressed. If your clothes are going to do the talking, though, make sure you know what you want them to say. Develop a personal style and then make it work for you. To paraphrase Heidi Klum, in fashion, one day it's in and the next it's out. Dos of yesterday are don'ts of today, and vice versa. The true science in this equation is your comfort. That being said, there are some basic fashion values that always equate in the common sense of putting yourself together.

In putting together a wardrobe that will get you through every situation, look for a few core qualities:

VALUE: If you invest in well-crafted clothes made from quality fabrics, they will last longer and serve you better. A bargain-bin purchase will probably fall apart within a year. Big-ticket, trendy items are generally a waste of money, since once they fall out of vogue, they'll only collect dust in the back of the closet.

CLASSIC DESIGN: Timeless designs will take you through decade after decade. Clean lines and simple cuts always complement a body more than excessive ruffles, puffy sleeves, or yards of fabric.

BALANCE: When wearing the right clothes, any body type can look great; the key is balancing your ensemble to create an even, uniform look. Wearing a baggy top with supertight jeans will only make you look like a trashcan on toothpicks. Prints and accessories also need to be in scale with the body.

BLACK AND WHITE: You can never go wrong with wonderful black and basic white; you can mix and match without a second thought. That's not to say color is a bad thing, either. The right colors can work magic. But if you are choosing color on a budget, think about the way black and white work, then try to build a monochromatic wardrobe so that you can combine different items and make use of all your favorites.

SIGNATURE STYLE: If you create a "signature" look, you'll always know how to look sharp, and people will remember you. Don't wear it every day, but use it as your go-to approach when you want to feel your most comfortable and chic. Think Sade, with her sleeked-back hair, red lips, and simple white shirts. Even Madonna, with all of her changing styles, has a signature approach for each period she is promoting. But be careful. You want to be remembered for your easy sense of style, not for looking "crazy" or "wacky." And you certainly don't want to get known as "that purple girl" or "the one with the weird hat."

OUT OF THE CLOSET

Want the quick answer to learning to love yourself more? Learn to love your closet more!

Your clothes are one of your primary means of expressing yourself, and if you are walking around in wrinkled, tired, out-of-style rags that you hate, you are going to have a tough time loving who you are. Most of us jam our closets so full we can't even move the hangers. We pile shoes on top of one another. We shove sweaters behind sweatshirts. Wrong! You should be able to see everything in your closet. You should be able to easily find that one item you need to make your outfit feel put-together. And you should only have items that make you smile when you take them out. Anything that makes you unhappy needs to go. So if you're a yo-yo dieter (and we'll get to that in the next chapter), put the "wrong" wardrobe into storage instead of torturing yourself with it.

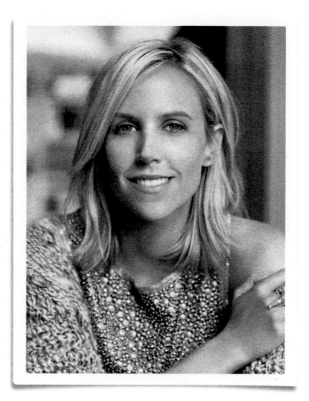

"Great style is knowing what you like and what looks good on you. It's about injecting your personality and what you love—whether it's bold color, mixing prints, or going for something totally sleek and minimal."

—Tory Burch, designer

Quick Challenge

Extreme Makeover:
Closet Edition

Take everything out of your closet and dresser drawers. Lay it all on the bed, arranging it by type (dresses, slacks, jeans, short-sleeved tops, long-sleeved tops, etc.). Now, slowly start to put everything back in the closet. Arrange each "section" by color, from lightest to darkest. Throw away anything that's worn-out and bag up anything you haven't worn in a year—it's going to the thrift store. Next, make a list of the basic items you feel like you're missing, and either start saving up to buy them or go shopping! Make sure you've got the ten following essentials covered:

1. ACCESSORIES: You don't need a treasure chest full of 'em, just a few choice baubles and bangles—necklaces, earrings, bracelets—to add a pinch of spice to your look when you need it. Again, "signature" pieces can go a long way.

2. BLACK DRESS: The basic black dress will take you from the office to the red carpet. Make sure it just covers the knee and fits you perfectly at the waist.

3. CARDIGAN: A soft wool or cashmere cardigan is perfect for year-round coziness and is appropriate in a whole host of situations.

4. JEANS: A pair of perfectly fitting, comfortable jeans can be dressed up or down. Hem them to wear with a pair of heels. Single-cuff them for flats.

5. SUIT: A well-made suit can get you through all kinds of situations, and also gives you two essential separates: a blazer and a pair of dress pants.

6. T-SHIRTS: You should have a V-neck, a U-neck, a square neck, a long-sleeved T, a short-sleeved T, and a tank. T-shirts are basic equipment.

7. WHITE BUTTON-DOWN SHIRT: A crisp, white button-down blouse will work with your suit or your jeans and can go formal or casual.

8. FLATS: A sensible pair of good-looking flats is a must. There's no need to always walk around in heels—any discomfort will be reflected in your face.

9. HEELS: Think simple and comfortable. Black is best for a first pair of pumps, since they will go with anything.

10. HANDBAG: Find your perfect bag, one that can hold all your on-the-go staples, and always have it at the ready.

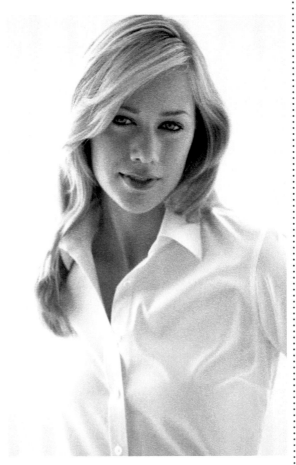

Rachel Minier

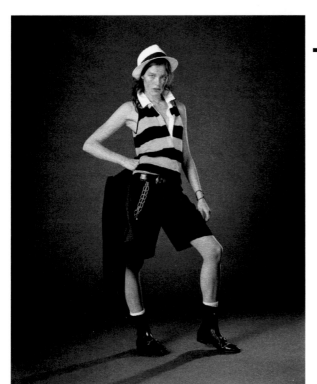

A FINAL WORD—OUTSIDE IN

What we have been talking about are the outer ways you can shine. Your image. Images are, literally, my business so, though I understand them, I also want to warn against them a bit. An image is an artifact, a two-dimensional picture; but you are a full-blown, three-dimensional person. The only way to choose the "right" makeup, hair, and clothing is to understand your total Beauty Equation. You can't look to others to define what you should wear any more than you can look to others to tell you who you are. Develop yourself and you will know what your personal style should be.

Lecture over! Now let's have some fun.

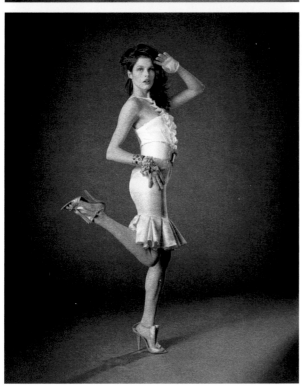

Lonneke Engel showcasing two different signature looks. Make it your own and go for it!

Skin-Deep: *the challenge*

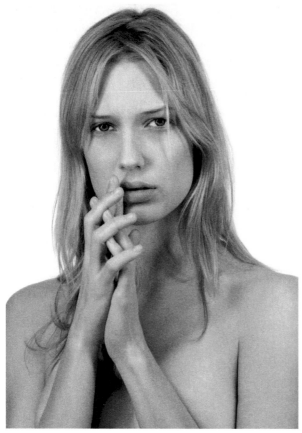

Sarah McNeilly shot for "the Art of Beauty" in *Tatler* magazine *au naturel*

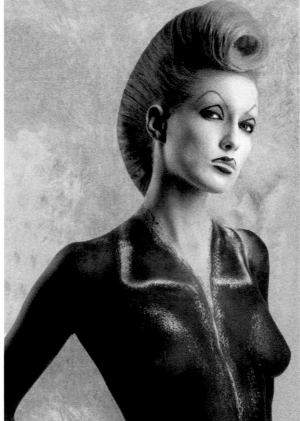

. . . and completely made over

1. NOTHING

Remove any makeup you're wearing and clean your face so you are 100 percent natural. If your hair is up, let it down. Wash any product out and let it fall where it may. Now, set your camera up to take a beauty shot of yourself—just your face. The only thing you are allowed to wear is a smile. Take a self-portrait!

2. A LITTLE

Now study your portrait from the previous challenge. What do you think is your face's best feature? Eyes, mouth, cheeks? Pull your hair up into a ponytail or a chignon. Take the one—only one!—feature you most like about yourself, and accent it with makeup. It might just be some lipstick. It could just be eye shadow. You're drawing attention to your greatest attribute. Now take a self-portrait!

How did the last photo come out? Were you able to convey your radiance with just a touch of makeup? Next, I want you to apply a face that gives you confidence. Use all the makeup you feel you'd need if you were coming in to see me for a shoot or heading to a special daytime event, say an outdoor wedding, where you wanted to look your best. Do your hair any way you like, but try and keep it off of your face. Wear a simple favorite outfit that you think flatters you, but don't accessorize yet. Try to bear in mind some of the tips we've discussed in this chapter. Take a self-portrait, a head shot, but also zoom back a bit and take another one to show off more of your look.

Compare the last shot to the first two. Do you feel the additional makeup has helped, or has it distracted from the way you look? What about your hairstyle and wardrobe? Regardless of the outcome, now I want you to really do yourself up. Have fun. Pretend you are going to a red carpet gala, an elegant scene where you will be photographed not only under dim lights but also under the bright flashbulbs along the red carpet. Do your hair so it looks its most glamorous and exciting. You can even dress up and accessorize. Take a series of self-portraits: close-ups, mediums, and wide shots. Show me all you've got.

Now, comparing these four setups, which one do you like the best? Which one says the most about who you really are? Which one says the least? Drawing from the strengths and weaknesses of these pictures, can you create an equation for your best basic look? Maybe even a "signature" look, one that will work at home, school, the mall, and a party? Play, and experiment. Try repeating the last three challenges and see if you get different results.

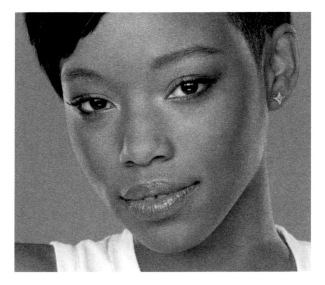

I hope that from now on, whenever you look in the mirror, you'll never ask, "Who's the fairest of them all?" Comparing yourself to others leads to jealousy and insecurity, two of the most unattractive qualities a person can possess. Your radiance has no peer. It is paramount to tend to how you look and present yourself, but the real glow comes from your inner fire. Remember, your beauty is not only skin-deep. It goes all the way to your heart.

Lulu Braithwaite, nineteen, aspiring model, capturing radiance

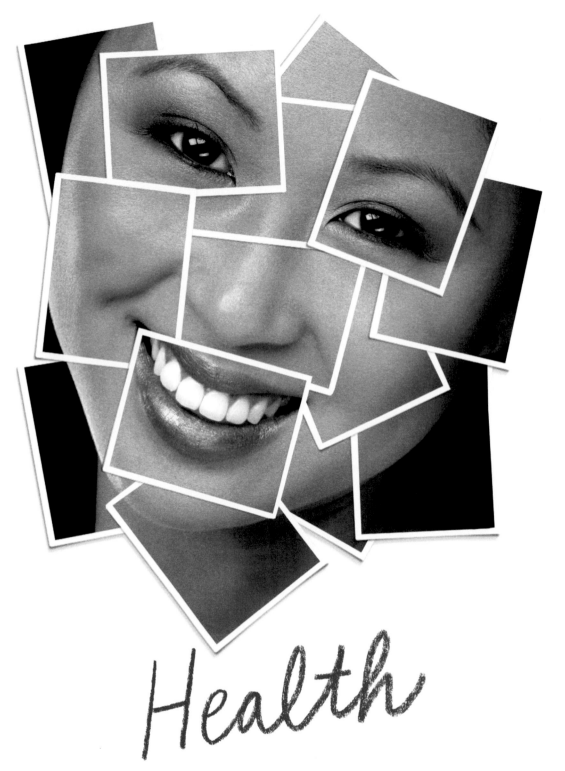

Health

TO BOOST YOUR VITALITY THROUGH BODY IMAGE

Skinny Bitch! Fat Cow!: *the teach*

STICKS AND STONES

Extra! Extra! Have you read the latest tabloid news? Who's got the best beach body this year? Is it Britney? Or is she "fat" again? It couldn't be Courtney, who is so thin she looks like a skeleton from a horror film. Did you hear . . . Angie fainted on set from lack of food! *Read all about it!*

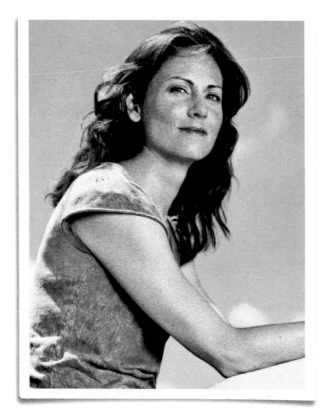

"Health is the foundation
to self-esteem. Healthy outlook,
healthy body, healthy influences:
They all add up to feeling
important, energetic and loved."

—Ave Shalom,
featured in *Health* magazine's "Real Health" tour

No matter how you slice it, the fashion and advertising industries have a furious obsession with body size, which encompasses both height and width. Women's bodies are used to sell everything from clothes to potato chips to diamonds to beer. This all-consuming concern with conforming to some precise body standard (which itself changes frequently) has trickled down through advertising, television, and the movies to make a national pastime out of sizing up not only celebrities in the public spotlight but also ourselves and those around us. "Look at that skinny bitch!" "OMG, she's a fat cow!"

OK, people, let's get back to common sense before we lose all sight of what truly makes for a healthy body. Ads are trying to sell products. Period. Trashy magazines and tabloid television news shows are trying to boost their own popularity by detailing the ups and downs of celebrities' relative happiness and public misery. Internalizing the stereotypes they promote and judging yourself and others by these manufactured industry standards is not good for your health. It only leads to a downward spiral of comparison and envy. Most women learn, through media distortion, to be dissatisfied with their personal appearance in some way, and that is just wrong.

We can all agree that advertisers currently champion an image of women who are superslim and impossibly tall. Why they choose an unattainable ideal to promote their product is beyond me and strikes me as just plain nuts. Isn't the whole point of advertising to say, "This product is attainable for *you*," and not, "This tall, thin woman couldn't possibly be you, but, um, buy this product anyway"?

Maybe the goal is to keep you in a state of flux so they are assured they can keep selling you diet bars and laxatives. Then the media further stokes the fire by constantly reinforcing that the women we love on-screen or in the fashion pages are too fat or too thin this week—when, often, the difference is only five to ten pounds. This constant brainwashing leads us to accuse perfectly healthy women in our own lives, who are neither too fat nor too thin, of being just that, shaming them into unnecessary self-doubt.

OK, we get it. Ads are trying to make us feel like we can brush up against the glamour a model projects by owning what the model is selling. And they're right: We love glamour. But we can't judge ourselves, our friends, our sisters, and our mothers against it.

Ultimately, the result of this constant nagging on the media's part is to keep real women in perpetual fear that they are in need of an adjustment, whether it be through fad diets, body shapers, or "miracle" creams. And the profusion of images of painfully thin models has the painful consequence of making real women's bodies invisible in media and advertising.

Been to Vegas lately? Every poor girl with a dream, dancing in a strip club to make ends meet, has fake breasts. Someone, somewhere sold them on the idea that it's sexy to have cantaloupes pasted onto your chest. Botox, lipo, skin resurfacing, nipping and tucking? Stop the madness. Look at yourself. Evaluate your body shape and make it as lovely as it can be through proper eating (notice I didn't say "dieting") and exercise. When it comes to inner beauty and projecting a positive self–body image, the advice here remains the same as throughout the *Beauty Equation*: Be yourself!

THE INDUSTRY STANDARD

In an attempt to standardize the fashion industry, the powers that be have created what is called a sample size. Designers create their clothing lines and construct all their garments in this one "perfect" size, size 6. Then, when it comes time to bring in the mod-els, they don't have to worry about the natural range of the human body. This standardization has nothing to do with the reality of the perfect size (since there isn't one) and completely ignores the fact that models aren't "perfect." No, not even models.

Of course, once designers have unveiled their sample apparel and it is approved, it will be manufactured in a range of sizes to fit real women. But while that process is in motion, designers choose to show their clothes to buyers on "fit" models, or human hangers. They are just the size designers are looking for and sometimes never even leave the showroom. You have never seen these models in magazines or walking down the runway, yet they are very much in demand and make a lot of cash. Because they are not in the ads or the public eye, they don't need to conform to age or beauty requirements. They only need to fit into the "perfect" size, a size that is not very common in the real world. But, personally, I tend to think clothes actually look better on a person than on a hanger.

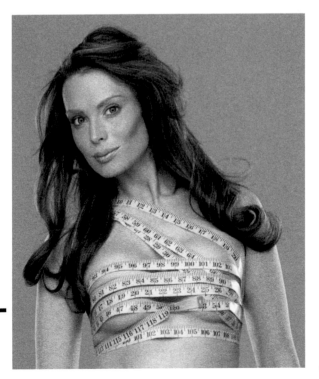

Yoanna House

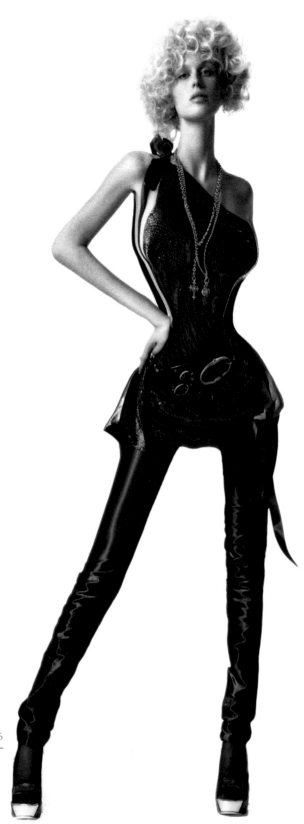

THE SKINNY ON SKINNY

Have you ever picked up a men's magazine and thumbed through the pages? Sure, there are articles on losing weight, but it is nothing compared to the weight-loss literature you will find in most women's magazines. Doesn't it seem like every other article aimed at women is promising you that if you just lose that ten pounds, the world will be your oyster and you'll have every man, woman, and child eating out of your hand? That if you could only look more like the model in the article, all your problems would magically disappear? Bull! Problems don't disappear with weight loss. Weight disappears with weight loss.

The pressure to be thin in this society starts to affect us from a very early age. Think of our Barbie dolls. If the popular doll were a real person, she would probably stand six feet tall, weigh a hundred pounds, and wear a size 4. She might suffer severe back pain from supporting her bust, and her body would be too narrow to contain a full set of organs, leading to some horrific consequences, which we are too polite to discuss here. A total fantasy, yet young girls aspire to be her every day—now *that's* a skinny bitch.

Unfortunately, in the United States, health has taken a backseat to the pursuit of "skinny." Girls start dieting as early as the first grade, and it is estimated that one in four young women uses an unhealthy approach to weight control. Skipping meals, excessive exercise, vomiting, and near starvation are not natural, nor do they lead to a fantastic figure. But sadly, *Teen* magazine recently reported that 50 to 70 percent of girls who are of normal weight believe that they are overweight.

I'm the first to agree that the fashion industry's glorification of ultraskinny models is unhealthy for young girls, who all too often aspire to be like them. However, there are millions of people who happen to have fast metabolisms and are naturally slim. We all know someone who says yes to the ice cream, the chocolate syrup, the whipped cream, the nuts, the sprinkles, and the cherry and never gains an ounce.

Caridee English, digitally manipulated to have proportions similar to Barbie's (hardly the Caridee we know and love, huh?)

> "Statistics show that most guys prefer skinny girls with cancer over healthy girls with bulging thighs."
>
> —Comedienne Gilda Radner, in her routine "Good-bye, Saccharin"

In fact, I know one very well: my wife, Crissy. The woman can eat like a horse, without consequence, while all I have to do is to look her way, and somehow I've put on weight! Well, believe it or not, my wife and her identical twin sister, Kimmy—who have both had successful modeling careers—often had problems booking jobs due to their size. They were too little. Coming in at a size 2, with delicate frames, they simply couldn't fill out the size 6 that most samples come in. They've always been two extremely healthy, beautiful women, inside and out. But it is nearly impossible, with their metabolisms, for them to size up, just as it's nearly impossible for many others to size down.

Quality, not quantity—that's what matters. Whatever your body type is, embrace it. Don't try to change it into something it isn't meant to be. Imagine winning a brand-new car in a raffle. Your ticket has been drawn and you are now the proud owner of a gorgeous Mustang! But when you stand up to accept your prize, you whine, "I wanted a VW Bug!" or "I pictured a Mini Cooper!" Your body is an amazing and beautiful prize. Don't cry about the model you've won and wish you had something else. Love it and learn how to drive it properly, and then cruise down the highway of your life with pride.

¡NO FLACAS AQUÍ!

In 2006, at the height of the "heroin-chic" era, with its waifish, bony models, Madrid, Spain, enacted the world's first ban on overly thin models at top-level fashion-show catwalks, during Fashion Week. Modeling agencies were outraged, claiming they were being used as scapegoats for eating disorders. But the boycott organizers claimed it was time for fashion to project an image of health and beauty, rather than emaciated glamour. In other words, they wanted to ban skinny girls from their runways, or, in Spanish, ¡No flacas aquí!

Spanish regional official Concha Guerra explained, "Fashion is a mirror, and many teenagers imitate what they see on the catwalk."

"I think it's outrageous. I understand they want to set this tone of healthy, beautiful women, but what about discrimination against the model, and what about the freedom of the designer?" said Cathy Gould of New York's Elite modeling agency. The move, she went on to argue, could harm the careers of naturally "gazellelike" models.

And what about the hombres? No one ever seems to be bothered by the guys. You rarely see tabloid headlines about Seth Rogen being too big or Taylor Lautner's chest not being muscular enough. When I was in my late teens and had just started modeling, I was in pretty good shape, but I had to work extremely hard to get there. I remember working with other male models who were in superb physical condition, yet they would come to set with boxes of chocolate and jumbo bags of chips and basically eat whatever they liked. Somehow, no doubt because of their genetics, they still had washboard abs. Should we also ban guys with washboard abs from advertising, as most young men will never acquire them and might spend years mentally beating themselves up trying to achieve them?

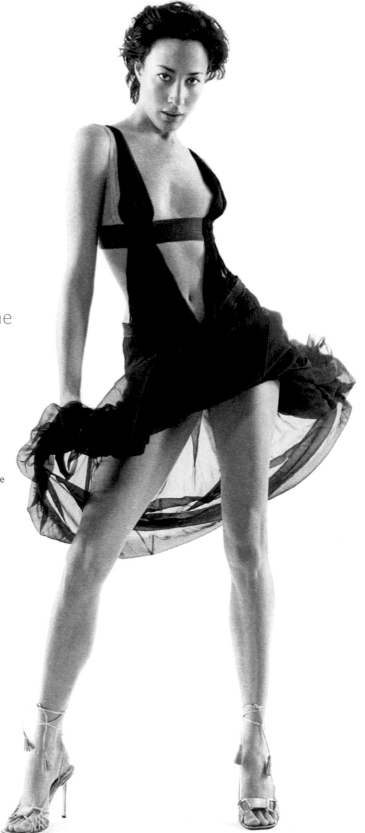

"I remember clients telling me I'm too thin to fit the clothes, while they would tell the girl next to me she was too big. The industry has this ideal girl they are trying to create. I had to learn not to take rejection personally. Most importantly, I did not want to change myself and be that ideal that clients expected me to be." —Kimmy Hise

ONE SIZE FITS ALL (NOT!)

There is no perfect size. We are all unique individuals and come in a variety of shapes and proportions. There's no shame in it. How boring would the world be if every woman were a "perfect" size 6? Also, just because the fashion and advertising industries have selected a type and size they think will appeal to the widest audience, does that mean they are always successful? Pick up any magazine. Now, start thumbing through the pages, stopping to look at every ad, every article, and most importantly, every picture of a person. Does every model who appears in an ad appeal to you? Is everyone "perfect"? Everyone is perfect in their own way, but that may not be perfect for you. We all have specific tastes. Just like there is really no one size that fits all, there is no measure of perfection in the human form capable of appealing to everyone.

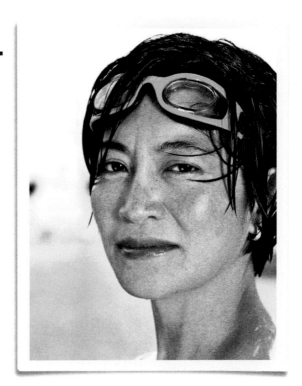

Quick Challenge
Who Is Perfect?

Grab a piece of paper and quickly jot down the five women and five men you think are as close to perfect as possible. They can be celebrities or people from your hometown. What is it you like about them so much? Is it pure physical beauty or is it that they crack you up? Are they wildly talented? When they sing, do you get little shivers? When they hit a tennis ball, do you find it exhilarating?

Once you create your list, upload it to www.beautyequation .com, under the "One Size Fits All (Not!)" forum. We'll conduct a little experiment and see just how many people are considered perfect. I'm sure it's going to be a massive list of names and will demonstrate that, although a lot of people find similar things attractive, we all have our own personalities and tastes.

"With good health comes the tools you need to have self-esteem—a clear mind and an active body. With just those two things, it is easier to feel good about yourself and, obviously, you are not relying on other people for your esteem."

—Tricia Foo-Ying, featured in
Health magazine's "Real Health" tour

MIND OVER MEDIA

What if I let the media tell me I wasn't worthy? What if I started to feel inferior to the men who were always hogging the covers of magazines? What if I started obsessing, thinking, "If only I had Brad Pitt's blue eyes," or "If only I had Josh Holloway's blond locks," or "If only I could rock a joke like Chris Rock," or "If only

I could woo my wife with a voice like Marc Anthony's" ... then I would be perfect.

I'd have to be kidding, right? If I really aspired to any of those goals, I'd be up the proverbial creek without a paddle. Why? Because none of those things are me. But just because I'm not blue-eyed or blond or a professional comedian or singer, that doesn't mean I'm not the perfect *me*. All I can ever hope to be is the best me. The only one in existence. If there were others, I would not be unique. And, by the way, my wife quite enjoys my singing (either that, or she is a very good actress).

I exercise on a regular basis and eat as healthfully as I can. I believe we should all do what we can to promote our own health. Health is the key to life and a prerequisite to any real success and achievement. In making "health" the goal (instead of "change") when exercising and eating, you will, ironically, bring about the most change—both in the way you feel and via your natural ability to radiate beauty. If you are working out and following a diet regimen solely to transform your body to meet some ideal, you have a hard row to hoe. It's very difficult to become someone else, someone you are not.

We all need to be mindful of how and what we eat, and whether we're getting enough exercise, whether we tend toward being large or toward being painfully thin. We need to treat our bodies with respect and not be too hard on ourselves if they don't immediately conform to our expectations. We need to be kind to ourselves, accepting our differences and celebrating our distinctiveness.

But we could all use a little help from the people setting the standards. That's why, as the fashion industry is slowly but surely starting to change, it's important for television and media to expand the public's notion about what is considered beautiful and to represent all demographics. All body types. All hair, eye, and skin colors. From short to tall, full-figured to stick-thin, always remember, variety is the spice of life!

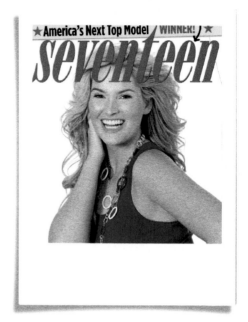

PICTURE OF HEALTH

WHITNEY THOMPSON

"I'm not emaciated, I'm not starving myself, and yet I'm considered plus-size. Why is that? Why is a healthy size considered too big?"

Truthfully, I don't think any model deserves the designation "plus-size." Most of the girls who are saddled with this label look quite normal to me. Yet, because of the industry standards, many girls with perfectly proportionate bodies are branded with it. Slowly, however, as advertisers learn who their consumer base really is, these "plus-size" models are growing in demand and getting more and more work.

Whitney is the picture of health. She has an incredibly positive attitude about life and her work. Making no excuses, she embraces her unique package and works it to full advantage, and it has rewarded her by taking her to the top. She is in constant demand because of her personification of youth, beauty, joy, and health.

Says Whitney, "I do feel good about myself, and I want other women in America to feel better about themselves. I honestly think that girls will look up to me and say, 'I can do that, I can be that.'"

GUILT IS NOT A PLEASURE

My wife and I have two children, Jack and Jasmine, and while Crissy bounced back to her former self since the births, I did not. Whether it is my changing metabolism or the fact that I kept her company for nine months in the "eating for two" campaign, I don't know. I have, as a result, tried many diets, only to reject them all. Instead, I've learned that I need to constantly be aware of what I put into my body and its likely effect. But that's not dieting. That's eating right.

Personally, I try to eat well not because I want to look perfect, but because I want to feel better and, hopefully, live longer. Although I found that certain food combinations work better than others at getting the weight off fast, when it came to keeping it off, I had to rethink my lifestyle. I didn't want to be constantly watching what I ate or abstaining, but I did need to work out what approach to eating would work for me. Turns out, I had to do very little. Everything in moderation, combined with regular exercise, was all it took. If you're eating a jelly doughnut every morning, that's going to cause some trouble, but indulge in one once in a while, and you're OK. When you label something as strictly off-limits, you're setting yourself up for failure. Soon you'll have entered the vicious cycle of feeling bad about yourself for "cheating," and—*poof!*—there goes your self-esteem, right out the window.

In short, set yourself up for success, not failure. You simply can't project beauty if you are walking around feeling bad about yourself.

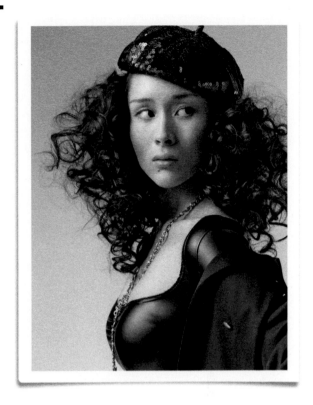

"Dark chocolate is my favorite guilty pleasure. I have a bar in my freezer at all times, just ready to go. I literally have a food-gasm when I eat it. I have it every day, so I never feel deprived. I balance that out by working my ass off at the gym. I work hard because I like to eat!"

—April Wilkner

"I never really bonded with my body. I just took it for granted, until I became a mother. While I was pregnant, I finally got the boobs and hips that I had always wanted, along with a big belly. Nature took over and I was in awe of what the human body was capable of: creating a life, nurturing it to grow, and feeding it once it was born. Our bodies are a gift that should be treasured and cared for. They may not always live up to our physical expectations, but we must respect their limitations and be happy for what we have."

—Crissy Barker

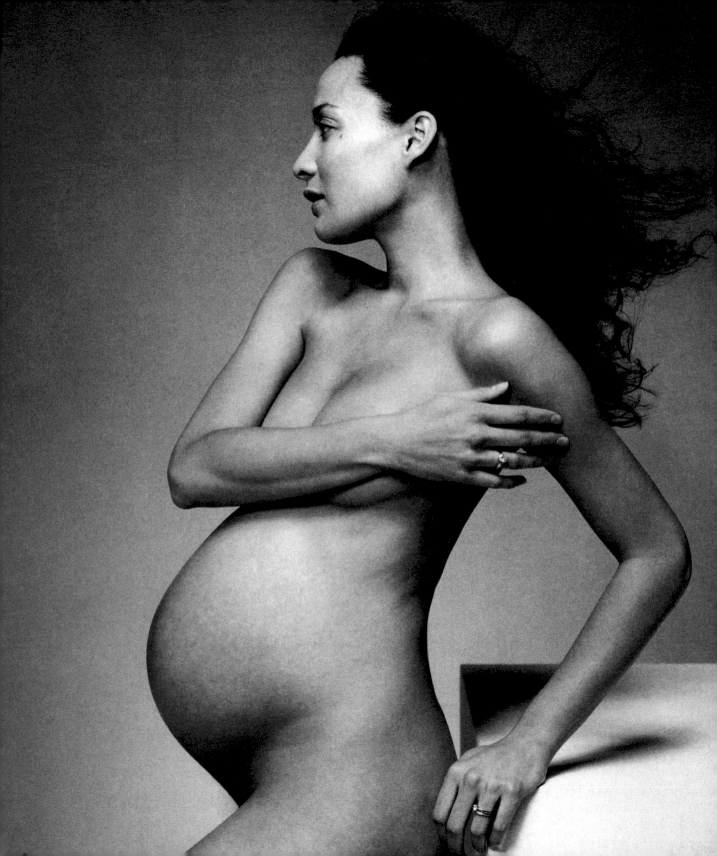

I'M NOT PERFECT
(BUT I WAS PERFECT FOR BASILE)

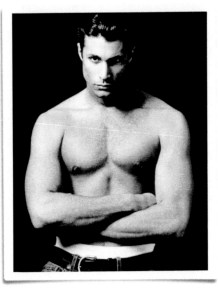

During my early modeling career

As we have discussed in previous chapters, confidence is key. In 1992, I was the model chosen to be the face of Italian designer Basile's advertising campaign. We shot the campaign without a hitch, but when I arrived in Milan to walk his fashion show, none of the clothes fit me. You see, I'm six feet four, which is really too tall to model most clothing—sample sizes come in a 40 regular, which fits a man of about six foot one. No amount of dieting or working out was ever going to change that statistic. Even worse, I was supposed to open the show wearing the suit I wore in the campaign. But instead of replacing me on the runway, the designer took a bold step. He simply tied the shirt and jacket around my waist and sent me down the runway bare-chested! Well, it caught the eye of the press and the public, making the statement, even if the clothes don't fit, you'll still want to drape yourself in them.

Basile's descision taught me an important lesson I've never forgotten. When it comes to business, you don't need the whole world to love you. You just need the person hiring you to get who you are, exactly as you are. One more trick: You have to believe in "who you are, exactly as you are," because in the end, you have to deliver.

There are many, many fad diets that come and go, always promising you the reward of weight loss if you just completely change the way you eat. No biggie, right? Ha-ha!

Diets that feature one primary food source, whether cabbage soup, grapefruit, apple cider vinegar, or acai berries, are all difficult to sustain but keep coming in and out of fashion. How can a single food really yield miracle results? Eating well is about balance, and when you tip the scales, there are sure to be consequences.

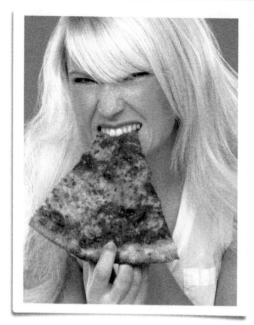

Alissa Laderer

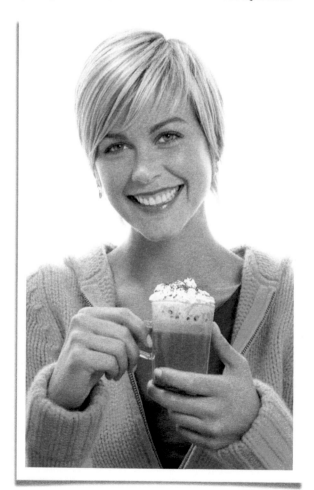

Rachel Cyriacks

There's the Zone, South Beach, Scarsdale, and Atkins diets, which all play with different combinations of carbohydrates, versus proteins, versus fat, versus your sanity. The problem with these diets can be that if you deviate from a very rigid set of rules, not only does the diet not work, but it can even backfire and cause you to gain weight and jeopardize your health. I'm not endorsing or dismissing any of these ways of eating. They all claim they work and have people who swear by them. If you do choose one of these diets, consult your doctor first to make sure it is right for you.

I do think that certain crash and fad diets can accomplish one good thing: They can force you, quickly, to break bad habits. You will definitely stop eating ice cream and french fries when you do the low-carb diets. You'll cut out red meats and fatty cheeses on the no-fat, low-cholesterol diets. And on both, you will learn to read food labels, which is incredibly important. The problem with any strict diet is that it holds you back from living life, which makes you miserable and stressed out, and that will never make anyone look beautiful, no matter how many pounds they shed.

THE GOOD, THE BAD, AND THE SUPER(FOODS)

Let's face it: Most of us can't afford to hire a personal chef in an effort to eat healthier, and we often only have time to grab a bagel or a candy bar when we're on the run. It's also difficult when you go to a dinner party or a catered event and the meal isn't particularly healthy (or even something you like).

While it's easy to let yourself slide and just take whatever looks the cheesiest, meatiest, or saltiest, bad eating takes its toll, both on your body and on the clarity of your mind. Here are some common-sense eating tips to help you make the healthiest choice, whatever situation you're in.

THE GOOD

Water, fresh fruit, and fresh vegetables are no-brainers. Train yourself away from other beverages and you will be craving water the minute you wake up, at lunch, and next to that glass of wine at dinner. Think about your desire for texture over your desire for a particular food item. Want something crunchy? Grab an apple or some nuts instead of that bag of chips or some other processed food snack.

THE BAD

Salt, sugar, and caffeine. This trio can do more damage than a bull in a china shop. Avoid adding salt to anything and, when you can, opt for sea salt instead of iodized salt (ordinary table salt not only has potentially harmful additives, but it has been processed and stripped of about eighty natural elements that still remain in sea salt). Don't overdo it on the desserts either, which often contain unhealthy amounts of both sugar and salt, and particularly avoid adding additional sugar to drinks, cereals, fruits, and sauces. Look, we all have a sweet tooth now and then, but bear in mind that sugar eats away at your teeth and nervous system and adds pounds rapidly. Small amounts of caffeine have been shown to have some positive effects, but too much can complicate body functions and become addictive. The worst offender of them all? Soda pop. Sodas are typically loaded with salt, sugar, *and* caffeine. In her book *Skinny Bitch*, Victoria Beckham describes soda as "liquid Satan." I don't know if I'd go that far, but I do think that if you care about your health, you should avoid it at all costs.

The minute you reduce your intake of these three criminals, you will begin to crave them less. A two-week personal sugar embargo will make a soda taste like the most overloaded, sugary-sweet food you've ever swallowed. And eliminate salt completely (even if it makes everything seem bland) for a couple of weeks and, before you know it, you'll start noticing the flavors of the actual food you're eating, rather than just tasting the added salt. Then, gradually, you can reintroduce it as it is meant to be used—in small amounts to enhance flavoring, not hide it.

THE SUPER

Look to the following "superfoods" regularly. They'll do wonders for your body and skin: almonds, apples, avocados, baked tortilla/pita chips, barley, blueberries, broccoli, brussel sprouts, cantaloupe, chicken (skinless), garlic, green tea, hummus, kidney beans, mackerel, oatmeal, olive oil, oranges, peanuts, pears, prunes, raw onion, salmon, strawberries, sunflower seeds, tofu, tuna, turkey (skinless), walnuts, and whole-grain muffins/bread.

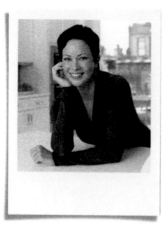

TOP TIPS FROM AN EXPERT

ELLIE KRIEGER

A registered dietitian and host of the Food Network's hit show *Healthy Appetite,* Ellie Krieger helps people achieve "beautiful" foods.

The best foods offer beauty from every angle. They are gorgeous to look at, they light up your taste buds with flavor and sensual pleasure, and they work from the inside out to help give your skin that priceless, healthy glow.

Foods like salmon—full of hydrating, skin-essential omega-3 fat; tomatoes, with their powerful, protective antioxidants lycopene and vitamin C; mangoes and carrots, whose brilliant-orange beta-carotene guards the skin from damage; even indulgent treats like high-quality chocolate and naturally sweet dried fruit have flavanoids that may improve skin's appearance.

But these foods aren't just good for your skin—they are good for every cell in your body. Your skin is the only organ you can see, and it is a reflection of what is going on internally. Beautiful outside equals beautiful inside. When you are healthy inside, you feel good, you radiate energy, and your eyes gleam. So fill your plate with these luscious foods and let your beauty shine through from the inside out.

EAT RIGHT, STAY FIT, DIE ANYWAY

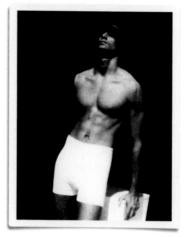

During my early modeling days

When my mom was a model in the early 1960s, the girls were far more petite and curvaceous than they are today—more along the lines of Marilyn Monroe. That matched up with her body type, so she got work. Then along came gorgeously unique Twiggy, with her boyish shape and mod haircut. Jobs for any other type dried up. Trends changed and my mother found herself working less. Still, she was the same beauty she always was. History repeated itself when I was modeling. It was the late eighties and the models were hearty, Amazonian. Apparently, I fit the bill. Then came the mid-nineties and the fashion industry, done with that fantasy, discovered heroin-chic, and the skinny, pasty grunge look took over. I realized that I was never going to fit into that mold and moved to the other side of the lens. Now, fitness is back in. So be it.

The point is, you simply can't ever try to make yourself over; you'll only end up a prisoner to the current trends. As Popeye famously said, "I yam what I yam!" What's "cool" today will be "over" tomorrow and, meanwhile, everyone travels the same path: birth, life, death. Make the most of it while you're here. Take care of your vessel and make it carry you as far as it can. Unless your goal is to be hired as a model, why should you care what's fashionable? What you should care about is whether or not you are exuding vitality, strength, spirit, and health—*life.*

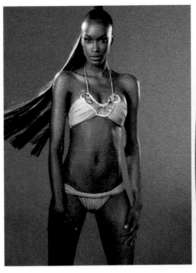
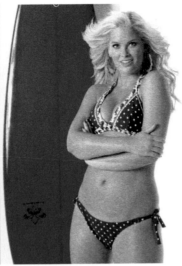

BODY TYPES
OVER THE PAST CENTURY

- **EARLY 1900s:** "The Gibson girl" was curvaceous, with a small waist and large breasts, a cartoon look that real women achieved by wearing a painful corset.

- **1920s:** Louise Brooks's showgirl look had little to do with fitness and more to do with style and personality. Compared to today's beauty standards, these lovelies were downright zaftig.

- **1930s:** High glamour was more important than body type—think Greta Garbo and Marlene Dietrich. Women didn't work out; they lounged on settees and drank martinis.

- **1940s:** The pinup girl tended to be leggy and full-figured à la Betty Grable and Lana Turner. Men in the war trenches dreamed of real girls with real bodies that they could grab ahold of on a cold, lonely night.

- **1950s:** Marilyn Monroe, Jayne Mansfield, and Sophia Loren set the ideal look. Exaggerated femininity, impossibly big curves. People wanted goddesses, not women.

- **1960s:** In an about-face in fashion trends, Twiggy's androgynous boy/girl stick figure took over as the standard. *Freedom* and *antiestablishment* were the buzzwords, and suddenly beauty was truly in the eye of the beholder.

- **1970s:** From Farrah to Fonda, women were fit but sexy, and girly or political. Black, Asian, exotic: Suddenly, it was anything goes. Women had come a long way and were ready to control their own image.

- **1980s:** Healthy, exotic, worked-out Amazonian girls-next-door ruled the runway. From Cindy Crawford to Naomi Campbell, it was survival of the fittest.

- **1990s:** Another 360-degree turn. Bored of the gym and ready to party again, heroin-chic beauties stormed the scene and waifish natural glamour was embodied in the image of Kate Moss. Suddenly every designer from Calvin to Prada wanted the look.

- **NOW AND THE FUTURE:** You tell me! What do you like and who do you want to see more of? My personal hope is that the era's renewed health consciousness will continue to influence advertising campaigns and magazine spreads to spotlight women who project inner beauty and real health.

ANTM winners Teyona Anderson (left) and Whitney Thompson (right), both healthy and fit, illustrating the fact that beauty comes in all shapes and sizes—waif, full-figured, and everywhere in between

BODY CONSCIOUSNESS AND CONSCIOUSNESS ABOUT BODIES

A good thing to keep in mind when you ogle the seemingly perfect lines of a model's body and smoothness of her poreless skin is that 99 percent of the time a retoucher has helped create that illusion. Retouching is now so commonplace that in Europe they are looking into legislation that would require all advertising images that have been retouched to say as much. Now, although that would burst the myth bubble over what is and what isn't retouched, you have to ask yourself whether the same rule should extend to makeup and lighting techniques too.

For millennia we have used makeup to both hide the way we look and emphasize the way we want to be seen. In the business of beauty, photographers and other artists use lighting and other tricks to flatter our subjects—to "blow out" or "soften" whatever we are hoping to disguise. So once again it boils down to common sense. Hopefully advertisers won't try to pull the wool over our eyes too much, but we do have to take everything we see with a grain of salt, understanding that there is artistic license at work.

Still, just because they are all "cheating" doesn't mean that you should too. In fact, you can't. That works in photography, in film, and on television. In real life, you have to walk into the room. You have to show up at the party. You have to shake someone's hand and be who you actually are. No Photoshop. No retouching. No postproduction airbrushing. No escape from the reality that you are standing there and have to be at your best.

A FINAL WORD— YES, YOU NEED TO EXERCISE

You don't have to work out twelve hours a day, but you do need to care for your body, tone muscles, create flexibility, and minimize whatever weaknesses you might struggle with. Not in pursuit of perfection, but in pursuit of health. Do it for no other reason than the simple fact that it will improve your Beauty Equation to have that extra glow.

Start with reasonable goals. Everyone says they don't have time, but who really doesn't have ten spare minutes a day for exercise? If the president of the United States can find time for it, so can we. Make it something that you know you can and will do. Like riding your bike to the store. Or volunteering to be the one who walks the dog. Dance around your room to your theme song. And once you're doing that one thing regularly, add one new doable exercise each week. Take the stairs two at a time at school. Park a block away from your friend's house and clench your butt as you walk to the door. Work up from ten minutes to thirty. Pretty soon, you'll be feeling more active. You'll want to maybe rent a yoga video or even go to the gym! Swim! Join a sports league! Wait a minute. Are you actually . . . exercising daily? You go, girl!

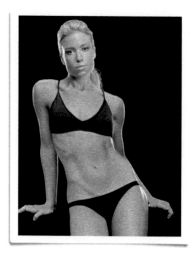

"This investment may be the most humbling struggle you have ever embarked on, yes, but the rewards are that it makes you glow and feel free. Getting good at regular exercise is not comfortable at the beginning. We have a universal responsibility to work smart and hard for our physical beauty."

—Tracy Anderson, celebrity trainer

Skinny Bitch! Fat Cow!: *the challenge* ☞ **BEAUTYEQUATION.COM**

1. QUEEN FOR A DAY

Treat yourself and your body! Pop out and get a manicure, pedicure, massage, or a facial. If a spa treatment is not within your budget this week, call a girlfriend to come over, and do each other's nails. The point is to reward your body for being so good to you. You love it and want to show it a little appreciation.

Now, take a photo of each part of your body: head, shoulders, arms, hands, thighs, calves, feet, and so on. The more specific the better. Add these to your online or printed portfolio and then finish the sentence, "This part of my body is beautiful because _____."

2. THE FINISH LINE

This is a four-part challenge, so get ready, get set . . . hold up. Before you get started on this one, an important thing to remember here is that you are looking to discover something new about yourself, not project some concept of perfection. A seasoned actor once told me that rehearsal is about discovery, not performance; that's why it's so important. These photos are for you to evaluate. Post them if you want to, but keep them private if that makes you feel safer. Now . . . go!

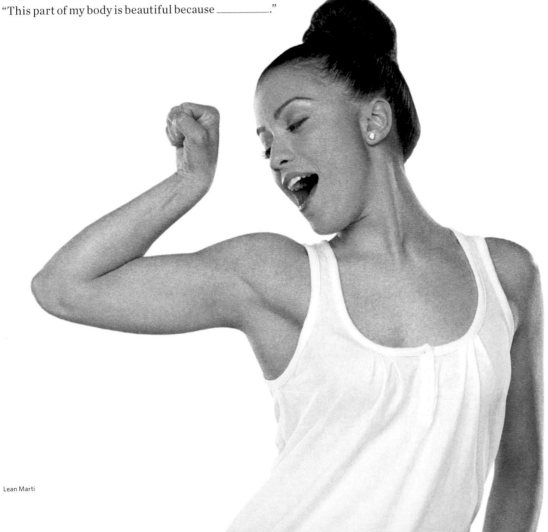

Lean Marti

- First, get dressed to work out, and take your initial picture. No makeup, no fuss.

- Next, you need to break a sweat. Whatever your sport or activity is, you're going to do it today. Run a mile. Bike to the beach. Aerobics, yoga, pilates. Doesn't matter. Just do your thing, but bring your camera so you can take your picture right after. Don't clean yourself up or try to look "pretty." You'll be sweaty and flushed, no doubt, but that's the point!

- Now, take a shower. Relax and try to let the postworkout glow shine through when you take your picture again, wet hair and all.

- Finally, get ready as if for a simple night out with close friends. Not too much makeup, no distracting clothing or accessories, your most natural hairstyle. Take one last shot to see if you can see any difference in your face as a result of today's exercise.

Comparing all four of these shots, you should be able to pinpoint what a bit of exertion does for the eyes, the cheeks, and even the way you hold yourself. Also, you should be able to evaluate whether or not you look great, in your own estimable opinion, right after working out, or if you clearly need a bit of time to recover. Overall, I'll bet you're surprised at how much good a little exercise can do for your look.

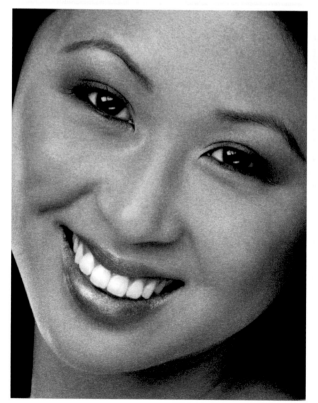

APPLES will always be apples and will never be oranges, and vice versa. One isn't categorically better than the other, but each has different benefits to offer, making one superior to the other only when you crave its specialness.

Comparisons are always damaging and rarely lead to a happy solution. Making a stand for who you are physically, mentally, and emotionally—as a unique person of the world with something to offer—with the understanding that there will always be people "better" and "worse" than yourself in any category is, in my opinion, a far healthier place to be. I like to think it is our imperfections that make us special. In this day and age, the world is a gorgeous melting pot with blurred bloodlines and cultures and we need to embrace that diversity, not conform to a single ideal of beauty. If there is a formula for beauty, then inner beauty is it.

Jami Kinton, twenty-five, dancer and reporter, capturing health

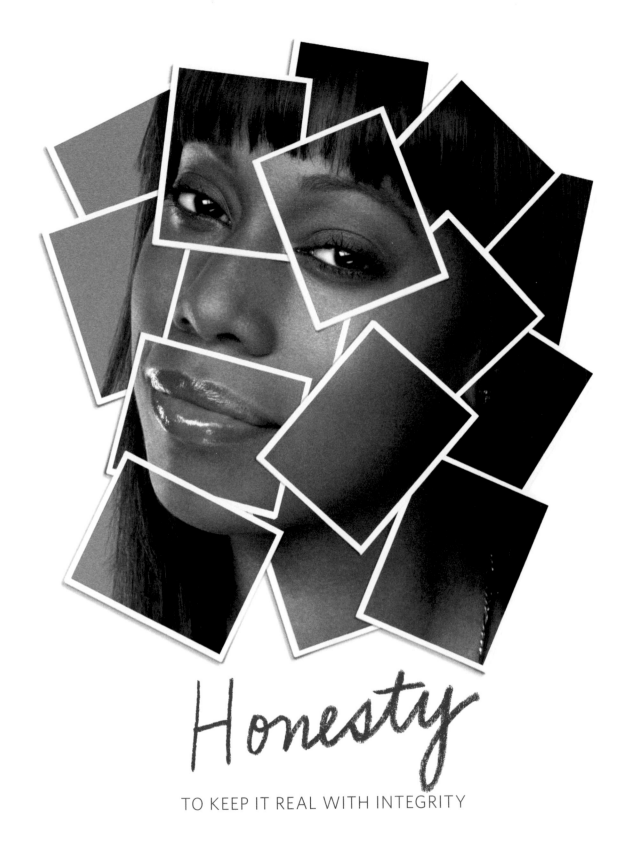

Honesty

TO KEEP IT REAL WITH INTEGRITY

> "The most natural beauty in the world is honesty and moral truth. For all beauty is truth. True features make the beauty of the face; true proportions, the beauty of architecture; true measures, the beauty of harmony and music."
>
> —Lord Shaftesbury

Beauty Lies in Honesty: *the teach*

HONESTY IS THE BEST POLICY

Have you ever heard the expression "The truth will set you free"? Know who coined it? According to the Bible, it's our common-language paraphrasing of some cat named Jesus. And do you know where the old saying "This above all: to thine own self be true" comes from? It's a line from a little play called *Hamlet*, written by a guy you might've heard of, Billy Shakespeare. People have been extolling the virtues of honesty for thousands of years, so there must be something to it.

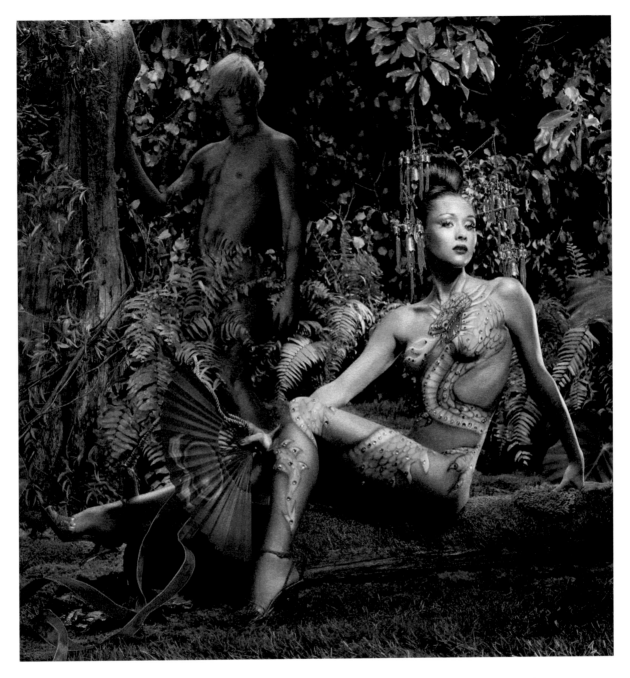

"Raw truth. Unapologetic, naked truth, whether in a film, a look, or a photograph, is so beautiful and inspiring. As a model and actress, I am most inspired when I see a subject let the audience see behind her walls and just let everything hang out. True beauty is flawed, original, and usually accidental."

—April Wilkner

Life is full of choices, and one of the greatest choices we face on a daily basis is whether to be honest with ourselves and with others. Consider this: How many times already today have you been asked a question or asked for your opinion? Maybe a waiter asked how your breakfast was. Maybe your friend asked you how she looked before she went out for the day. Maybe your boyfriend demanded, "Who ate all the chocolate-chip cookies?"

And how did you answer? Are you always able to answer honestly from your heart, or are you prone to squeeze the truth because you're a nice person? Would you tell your waiter, "Well, actually, my eggs were cold and the bacon was soggy," or would you smile politely and say, "Everything was fine"? Would you tell your friend if her eyeliner was crooked or she had lipstick on her teeth, or would you give a cheery grin and just say, "You look great! Go for it." And where *did* those delicious cookies disappear to? Would you 'fess up, or would you keep your late-night binge to yourself? Choices, choices.

In my experience, coming into contact with as many people as I do every day, I find the problem is keeping track of where the truth begins and ends. There's nothing worse than getting that puzzled look from someone when you contradict yourself. "But yesterday you said . . ." And then you scramble, trying to remember what it was that you *did* say yesterday. How awful is it to be out-and-out caught in a lie? There is nothing so pathetic as trying to backpedal your way out of one.

Honesty is a virtue, as they say, a character trait or quality that is valued in society. But life happens, so staying honest at all times is indeed a difficult battle. White lies (like accepting a hideously ugly gift with poise) are a necessary part of life, used to spare feelings, to benefit friends and colleagues, save relationships, ease hectic situations, or buy ourselves time in a crisis. The goal is to never allow yourself to be thoroughly untruthful—to act from honest intentions—as often as possible. Honest people gain the trust of others. They are *trustworthy* and genuinely likable.

Want to lose friends and allies? Lie. Want to be seen as indelibly essential to others, in love and elsewhere in life? Act from your best and most honest intentions, and people will know they can rely on you. Pretty women may lie, but beautiful women always tell the truth.

Being an honest person means you have staying power—that's why it's part of your Beauty Equation. Think about it: We might fall in love with someone for any number of reasons, but we stay in love with someone because they are honest and we can trust them. You can withstand almost anything from someone you love, but a break in trust makes relationships fall apart.

FROM "HONEST ABE" TO "TRUTHINESS"

We've all heard the tale of George Washington cutting down a cherry tree with his new hatchet and, when confronted by his father, owning up to it with the legendary, "I cannot tell a lie." Historically, up until the national crisis over Nixon and Watergate changed our perceptions forever, American presidents were legendary for their honesty. Abraham Lincoln even earned the nickname Honest Abe for his ability to stick to his guns and always tell the truth.

Today, we almost categorically accept that our leaders lie, cheat, and steal behind the scenes. In fact, public opinion polls suggest that we actually think they need to in order to survive the cutthroat world of backroom politics. We even have a new word for it. Coined by comedian Stephen Colbert, *truthiness* describes statements made by politicians and members of the media, without regard to evidence, logic, intellectual examination, or fact. It was even named Word of the Year in 2006 by Merriam-Webster!

It may be funny, but the message behind it is pretty frightening. The further the culture moves away from the virtue of honesty, the harder it is to remember how crucially important it is, especially in our own lives.

I have to make tough decisions and give my honest opinion all the time on whether I think someone is right for a job, has what it takes, or has potential. Unfortunately, the honest truth is not always nice to hear. Of course, giving your honest opinion requires that you are being honest with yourself in the first place. If your opinion is built on misconceptions and skewed truths you've built up to suit yourself, then your honest opinion is not going to be worth anything to start with.

America's Next Top Model, along with *Survivor, American Idol, The Amazing Race, The Apprentice, Big Brother, Dancing with the Stars,* and *Fear Factor,* is part of a new wave of reality television that first made a global impact in the 2000s. But having been a part of this groundswell of popularity, I can tell you that "reality" television is not always real. Many of the contestants on the shows I've mentioned have publicly proclaimed they were not portrayed in a true light. Many reality stars believe the TV audience doesn't get to see who they really are or the real situations that they were a part of. Well, I'm here to tell you something that may surprise you. Shows constantly cut out the appallingly bad behavior of their contestants so viewers won't just turn off the set. (Of course, it is also true that through a similar process of selective presentation—because it makes for better drama and higher ratings—some jerks come off as nice, and a number of lovely people come off as dorks.)

If you do watch reality shows you know that the most disheartening thing a contestant can do is change personalities before your eyes. When you trust someone, and then they boldly reveal to you they are a liar or a cheat, everything goes down the drain. For you to like someone for what they appear to be requires faith and trust. If someone betrays that, you become filled with doubt and uncertainty. Not a good formula for a successful Beauty Equation.

I have a friend who says we are drawn to reality TV because it represents a "microcosm of the macrocosm" of human behavior. It's an interesting theory. If we look at behavior on reality TV as representing small worlds (microcosms) that enlighten us about the whole of humanity (macrocosms), we see that contestants may get ahead by being dishonest, but, in general, when they betray alliances, and lie to each other's faces, steal from other contestants, or disrespect their property, knowingly sabotage them, or engage in mean-spirited behavior at their expense, they tend to lose votes among their panel of peers. Not to mention the audience at home.

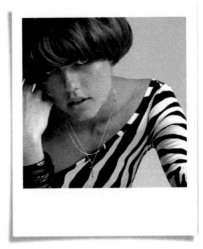

HONESTLY ME

KIM STOLZ

"To me, true beauty means being honest, having a confident opinion, not being ignorant, and being exactly who you are, regardless of others' judgments. As a gay person, I have encountered some obstacles over time with regard to my sexuality, but the one thing that has always gotten me through and kept me feeling beautiful was being myself and loving who I wanted to love, despite what it sometimes seemed society wanted me to be."

Kim Stolz is one of the most honest and fun women I've had the pleasure of watching on reality television. And as is clear from her TV appearances as an openly gay person, Kim is completely forthright in who she is as a person and a model. She never compromises her integrity. And as a result, she remains a remarkable and memorable character.

Kim's honesty about herself is an undeniable asset. A fearless competitor, she is able to deliver on whatever challenge gets put before her. And because she is so at ease with herself, she always has a blast. She is constantly entertaining and never at a loss for words. Why? Being yourself means you can soar. You never have to think twice or scheme for an excuse. You just are.

Take it from Kim: "Just be yourself. It might not feel like it's working right away, but it truly is the path to success."

TO BE HONEST . . .

Let me confess something to you. I prefer women with nothing on. That is to say, when I shoot a woman's portrait, I like her wearing no makeup whatsoever. Think of soft, simple lighting that reveals all without accentuating anything. The real you—the face that only you get to see most of the time. No hiding behind fake eyelashes, layers of foundation, or tons of powder, with all manner of shading and contouring. That's not to say there isn't a time and a place for that kind of thing, as of course I am well aware that a skilled makeup brush can do wonders. I just love the natural look the most, because it betrays such unavoidable honesty from the subject.

When professional models come to me on go-sees, it's almost unheard of for them to come "made up" (of course, they become very good at applying light makeup that accentuates their best features in a way that is hard to notice). It's vital for me to see them this way; otherwise, I simply can't evaluate what they look like. And you may be surprised, but I always think they look much more attractive with less or no makeup on—honest, real beauty.

How often do you wash the makeup off your face and examine yourself in the mirror? No doubt for a minute or two in the morning, and perhaps at night on your way to bed. And I imagine you feel you're being honest with yourself when you let that unkind inner voice say things like, "I hate my face without makeup." Well, if my assessment is correct, I suggest you spend a little more quality time in front of the mirror getting to know yourself without your war paint. Honesty isn't being unkind—it's being critical in the nonnegative sense of the word. Being *critical* about something means that you are critiquing it, good and bad.

Stare into your own eyes. Get lost in them. Watch your lips open and close. Tilt your head in different directions and pick your best natural angles. Smile. Frown. Grin. Smirk. Imagine my camera loving that you have no makeup on. Try to drop all pretenses and gaze at the honest reflection there, looking back, feeling exposed. There's no one there but you and your amazing, one-in-a-million face. Beautiful.

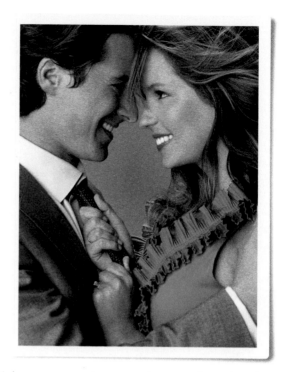

"I love wearing makeup that looks natural because it lets my true self shine through. I also believe transparency and honesty are fundamental attributes of a healthy relationship. My husband and I are completely honest with each other and have an open line of communication, and I think that enhances our love and trust for one another"

—Eleanor Langston, beauty director, *Fitness* magazine, with husband, Bradley Langston

137

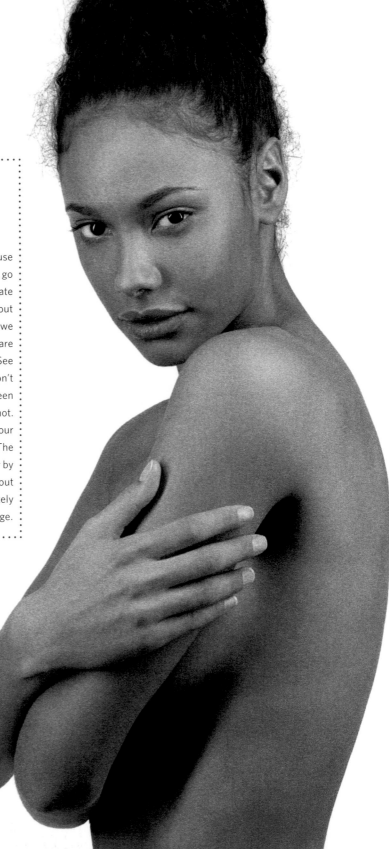

Quick Challenge
Bare Naked Beauty

Are you one of those women who never leaves the house without your full makeup on? If you are daring enough, go out barefaced, letting everyone see the real you, to evaluate how people in your world react differently to you without your usual mask. I know it's intimidating, and sometimes we have blemishes that we're embarrassed about, but these are things that don't or shouldn't define who we are, right? See what people say, and note the way in which they look (or don't look) at you. If you usually wear lots of makeup, you've been saying something to the world, whether you know it or not. It's not necessarily good or bad, but makeup changes your face and communicates things without your realizing it. The point of this experiment is to see if you are surprised either by people's new reactions to you or by your own feelings about yourself. You might not get an "answer," but you'll definitely gain awareness about makeup and its bearing on your image.

Tatiane Carvalho (left) and Azura Vandenberg

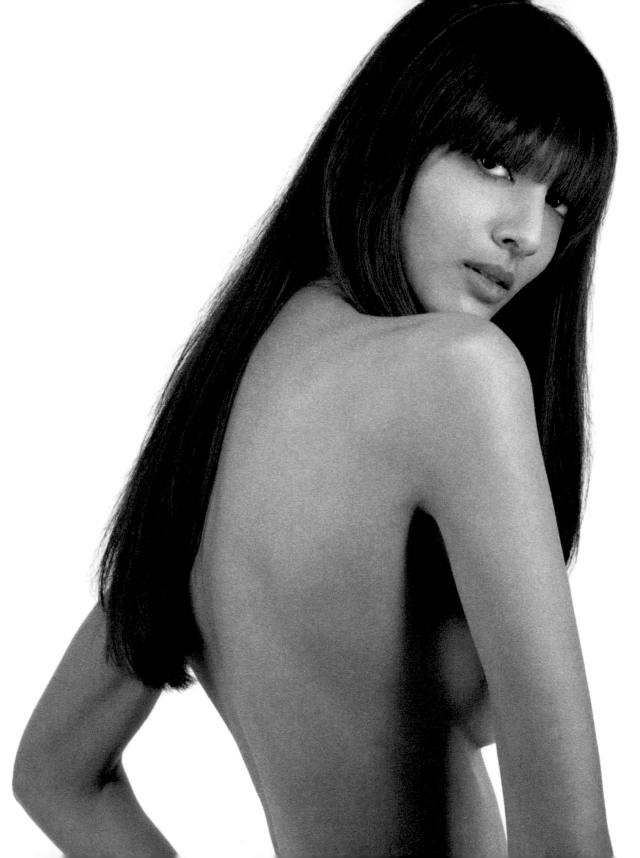

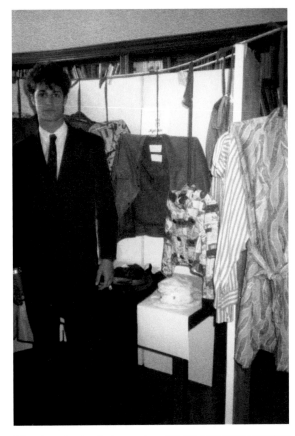

At Bryanston, my boarding school, age seventeen, with clothing I had designed, sewn, and won a school prize for (the first boy to win in that category)

As a young man I was good academically in the sciences, so it seemed like I was destined to be a doctor of medicine. But my heart lay in the arts. I was happiest reading English prose, studying art history, and basically, making things, whether it was taking photographs, carving wood, welding metal, or designing clothes. Still, I applied to medical school as seemed expected. Then, at age eighteen, fresh out of boarding school, I was cajoled by my mom into entering a modeling competition on a popular British TV program called *The Clothes Show*. It was a lot of fun and opened up a whole new world for me. I decided to take a year off to pursue modeling before going to college. Before I knew it, one year led to two—and the rest is history. Suffice it to say that I followed my heart, and by being honest with myself about what I wanted, I managed to create a life in which I've had few regrets. I fear that, had I taken a different path, I would be telling a very different story.

Occasionally, when I am casting or interviewing new talent, I feel like I am being told what they *think* I want to hear. While that can be very flattering for me, it can also be very dangerous for the girl on the hot seat. At an interview or your own life's "auditions," you only have a couple of minutes to get your potential across, and believe me when I tell you that honesty pays off. How you deliver the truth matters too, of course, but in any situation, if you lie to get ahead, you'll only have to dig yourself out later.

Case in point: I was shooting a job for a magazine that required the models to wear bikinis and get wet. The magazine editor cast the job and booked a stunning brunette, whom I only met on the day of the shoot. We were at a gorgeous, stately home out on Long Island, New York, and when I asked the girl to dive into the pool, she promptly said she was four months pregnant and didn't want to. Well, I improvised and still got a workable story, but I felt like we had been deceived into hiring her. Although I sympathized with her position, out of principle I never booked her again.

WE'RE ALL IN THE SAME BOAT OR *WIR ALLE IM GLEICHEN BOOT*

OK, since we're being honest here, I, of course, am guilty of telling half-truths too. As a young model I went to a casting where they asked me to fill out a questionnaire about myself. In high school I had taken French and German, so I ticked various boxes on the questionnaire suggesting this. I never thought that I would get booked for a TV commercial, sight unseen, requiring me to recite a script in Swiss German! Luckily, when I turned up on set in Austria for the commercial, the model I was working with was able to phonetically spell out my script and help me through it. The whole while I was terrified that I was about to get busted. I guess you could argue that it was worth ticking those boxes (I got the job and got through it), but my discomfort in the situation actually taught me a life lesson: Never overstate my current abilities.

Don't let yourself down. If you go about your business or your everyday life kidding yourself about what you have achieved and what needs to be done, you'll never actually get anywhere. People are constantly asking me, "Could I model? Do I have what it takes to work in the industry?" And sometimes I think to myself, "Really? This five-foot-two girl believes she has model potential? Does she fully understand that the odds are against her? Is she prepared for all the extra work she'll need to put in?" It's not necessarily that I doubt she can do it, but that it's going to be that much harder for her.

Millions of us enjoy the voyeuristic thrill of watching *American Idol* auditions on TV, and marvel over how these people can truthfully believe they can sing. And then we think, "Come on! They're pulling my leg! They just want to be on TV!"—until they start to cry and scream obscenities when they don't get chosen for Hollywood Week. *Same concept.* The self-deception is provocative (and ratings-grabbing) because we identify with it. We all fear being clueless sometimes, and the comic relief feels good because we're generally pretty hard on ourselves. Again, being honest with yourself doesn't always mean being tough on yourself. Instead, think about it as truly loving yourself for who you are and what you are. Only by assessing the areas where you are "challenged," along with loving your actual assets, of course, are you really being honest with yourself—and letting your true beauty shine.

(DOWNLOAD)

SONGS ABOUT HONESTY

*"Honesty is hardly ever heard.
And mostly what I need from you."*

"Honesty" —BILLY JOEL

"True Colors" —CYNDI LAUPER

"Respect" —ARETHA FRANKLIN

"True" —SPANDAU BALLET

"Tell It Like it T-I-Is" —THE B-52'S

SONGS ABOUT . . . DISHONESTY, DECEPTION, DECEIT, AND THEIR EFFECTS

"Lies, lies, lies (they're gonna get you!)."

"Lies" —THOMPSON TWINS

"Criminal" —FIONA APPLE

"Liar, Liar" —DEBBIE HARRY

"Smooth Operator" —SADE

"You're No Good" —LINDA RONSTADT

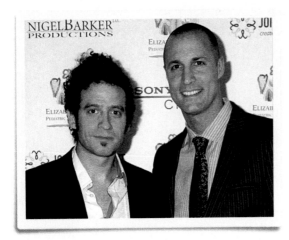

With Marcus Brooks

HONESTLY, I'M NOT GAY!

And then there are the various shadings of truth, which can make for some funny moments. One of my assignments took me to China. I was given a large duplex suite in the hotel in Shanghai and, as I wasn't traveling with my family, Marcus, my trusty photography director and close friend, stayed with me, sharing the suite. On the first morning there, we went to the hotel concierge to ask about sightseeing in the local area, and he asked us whether we were both staying at the hotel. We answered, "Yes, we're both staying in . . . a suite . . . um . . . at the hotel" (i.e., the same one!). When we eventually made a dinner reservation with him, he asked for our hotel room numbers and we had to come clean. We gave him the number to the room that we shared, to which he wryly remarked, "Ahhhh, two men in one suite . . . (wink, wink, nudge, nudge). Say no more . . ." (Being gay in China was illegal until 1997 and classified as a mental disorder until 2001.) Suddenly the obviously gay staffers at the hotel were all saying hello, smiling, and being extra nice to us, as it was still a touchy subject for Chinese men to be out. The moral being that, although we both told the truth in that we were indeed staying in "a suite," we were both being dishonest enough to make his mind wander, trying to figure out what we were trying to hide. Dishonesty changes people's perception of you and encourages them to fill in the blanks.

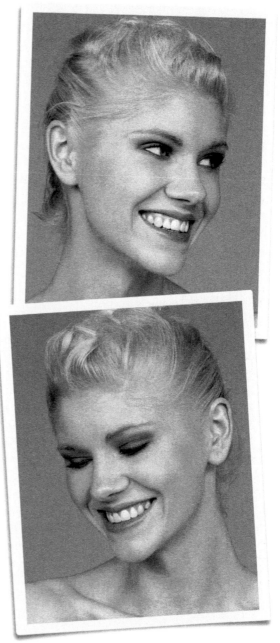

"Instead of telling a white lie, you can always answer with a suggestion and skirt it. As long as you leave that person feeling confident, then that is all that matters."
—Rebecca Epley

THREE WAYS TO IMPROVE YOUR HONESTY QUOTIENT

1. FOR A WHOLE DAY, TELL NOTHING BUT THE TRUTH

No white lies, no withheld information, no fudging the facts. At home, at work, at the supermarket, and everywhere. It's hard! Most of us would never be able to do it every day, but trying it will enlighten you as to the areas in your life where you are not being completely honest with yourself and others.

2. REVEAL A SECRET TO SOMEONE

We all have them! Pick someone you trust and tell them something no one else knows about you. Chances are, you'll feel like a weight has been lifted off your shoulders, and you might even find yourself unburdening more than you originally expected to.

3. MAKE A LIST

Put down all the people you were once close to that you have lost touch with. Why did the friendship fizzle? Is your list long or short? Were there trust issues? Here's a tough question: Could it be that some of those issues stemmed from you?

A FINAL WORD— HOME IS WHERE I WANT TO BE

In order to succeed in both business and life, you need your colleagues, friends, and loved ones to know that they can trust you (and vice versa). I give huge credit to my wife when it comes to my own success. We trust each other implicitly, and by that I mean that because we love each other, we don't let dishonesty or jealousy get in the way. I am frequently asked by interviewers whether my wife is jealous of me working with loads of pretty girls and traveling to exotic locations. The answer is no. Honesty is a cornerstone of our relationship, and we both know that we love each other. Of course, I do work with a lot of pretty girls and I do travel frequently (alone—except when I'm with Marcus, of course!), but I am never happier than when I am at home.

For me, being at home is being with someone I trust, and someone who trusts me enough in return to feel secure when I go out and do what I love to do. Whatever it is that feels like "home" to you, be sure to recognize it, be thankful for it, and never take it for granted. Carrying a strong sense of what it means to be at home will embolden your ability to go out into the world projecting the beauty that comes from honesty, trust, and strength.

1. ANDY WARHOL'S SCREEN TEST

In the 1960s, American artist Andy Warhol made the legendary prediction, "In the future, everyone will be famous for fifteen minutes." With the rise of reality television and YouTube, his prophecy has in many ways come true. When people would visit Warhol in his studio, he would often ask them to do a "screen test." He captured upwards of five hundred people in front of his tripod-mounted 16mm camera, asking them to stay as still as possible and telling them not to blink while the camera was running. It was actually an art project where the idea was that a person's honest self couldn't help but be revealed. "You look at a camera for so long, and what happens is that finally your true personality just leaps out, because you can't hold your pose anymore," said actress Mary Woronov, one of Warhol's factory "Superstars" (members of his clique whom he promoted as if they were celebrities).

Now, try it for yourself. Set up your video camera and tape yourself for five minutes. Stare into the lens and try not to move or blink. It will be the longest five minutes of your life! When you are done, watch the video, studying your face and your honest reactions. What does your screen test reveal about you?

2. THE TABLES HAVE TURNED

Think about who you trust the most. Is it your best friend, your mother, a sibling, maybe your boyfriend? Make a date for them to come over. Make sure the two of you can be alone. Now, shake hands with your guest photographer and photo director for this challenge. You are going to hand the camera over to them. Tell them how much you trust them and value their opinion.

Don't make any suggestions or reveal anything you have discovered about yourself and your honesty. Just tell them to take your picture in the way they think you are most beautiful. Let them decide how you should wear your hair, how your makeup should be done, and what kind of lighting they want to shoot you in. Now, have some fun!

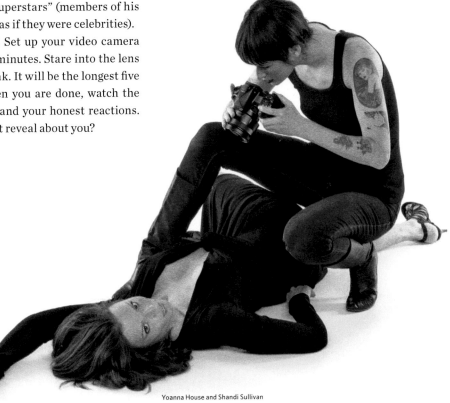

Yoanna House and Shandi Sullivan

144

Make some popcorn for yourself and your trusted one. Tell them to get ready to "make like Nigel" by following up after working with you on the photo shoot and helping you choose what pictures should go before the proverbial judging panel. You two are going to pore over your film to find the "selects." Study every portrait your steadfast photo director has taken and analyze each one. What about these photos do they find beautiful? Which of the photos do you both like best, and why?

Bear in mind that trust and loyalty are some of the most endearing gifts one person can give to another. Showing appreciation to those you love will not only strengthen the relationship you share, but will also bring both parties happiness. Thank them for their time and their honesty!

When your photo director leaves, add the pictures they chose to represent your honest beauty to your online or printed portfolio. Write a brief sentence or two about what each picture says to you. Was there something your confidant brought to light that you hadn't seen before or something that revealed an element of your Beauty Equation you hadn't thought of?

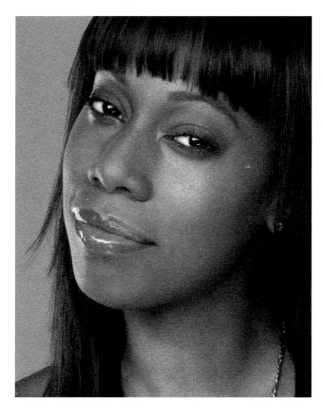

TO really succeed at anything at the highest level, you have to put your heart into it. If you don't believe in what you are doing or have the conviction to make hard decisions, you're not going to be able to follow through. It's so important to listen to who you are and understand what you need. In the modeling industry, girls are always being asked to be someone else, to act or perform, and of course the most successful models aren't always the prettiest, but rather the ones you believe in. The models that can sell you an emotion like happiness or sex appeal, because it appears to be emanating from them like raw talent. We all have this in us; some of us just need to gain the confidence to pull it off. Remember, the truth will set you free!

Mercedes Andrews, twenty-two, receptionist, capturing honesty

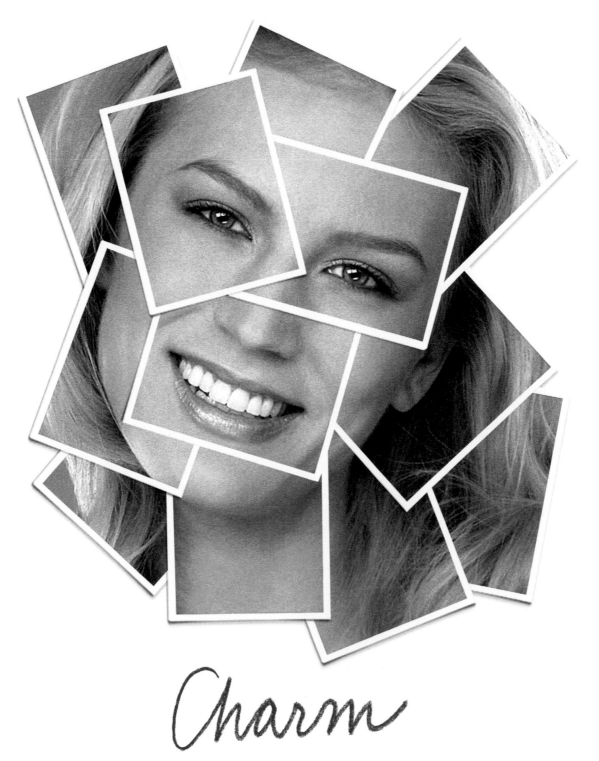

Charm

TO MAKE YOUR PERSONALITY SPARKLE, WITH WORDS

> "Charm is a way of getting the answer yes without asking a clear question."
> — Albert Camus

Oral Assault: *the teach*

LUCKY CHARMS

Don't you hate the new Millennial corporate sales training that programs the supermarket checkout cashier to ask you every time without fail, in that flat, disinterested monotone, if you "found everything you were looking for today?" Or the dead-eyed salesgirl at the clothing outlet who reads your receipt before handing it to you, seemingly in a concerted effort to mispronounce your name, as she says, "Thank you, Miss Blahdeblah. You saved three dollars today." A friend of mine calls this new brand of hypnotized trainees "the Zombies of Voodoo Island," suggesting they'd been shipped off to some faraway land where they were robbed of all charm in order to come back and better serve us with their "customer service." Their utter lack of charisma makes me want to run from the store screaming, abandoning my packages and just hoping to make it home safely without being lobotomized along with the rest of them.

No matter how devastatingly gorgeous someone is on the outside, when they open their mouth to speak and something unspeakable comes out . . . the interview, the date, or any hope for magic is over before it's begun. People completely underestimate just how powerful and persuasive they can be by applying simple, elementary charm.

British psychologist Havelock Ellis characterized charm as "the power to effect work without employing brute force," adding that it was indispensible for women. It almost sounds like magic, doesn't it? And a truly charming person is sort of magical. So what is this elusive quality? And what are the elements of charm that are so integral to the Beauty Equation?

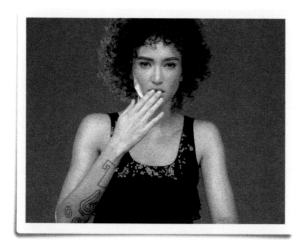

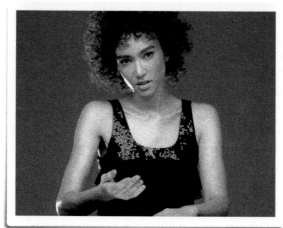

Naima Mora signs, "Thank you"

The charming Rachel Smith, Miss USA 2007, shot in New York's Meatpacking District

Whether holding the door for someone or just uttering the two easiest expressions in the vernacular of courtesy, "please" and "thank you," you can win hearts and minds. But it all depends on how you do it—how you sound and what you really feel. If you hold the door for one person at the bank and a line of folks seize the opportunity to take advantage of your kindness, and then you roll your eyes and say, "Who do you think I am, the doorman?" well, then the whole gesture is lost. The same is true if your delivery of "please" and "thank you" is merely a robotic response and you don't really care one way or another. Did you actually look at that person you were asking "please" of? Had you already turned your back and started to walk away when you muttered, "Thanks" to the barista for making your to-order latte? Your words are your connections to the people around you. If you are talking without thinking, you're not connecting.

The thing about charm is that it's empowering. When you float through life not giving a damn about those around you, you don't grow—and you certainly don't captivate. You don't need to get a gold star every time you do a good deed. When you mean what you say and say what you mean, though, you do get put on a pedestal—inside. And meriting that inner, personal reward increases your ability to enchant others exponentially.

Gratitude and grace, as important as they are, however, aren't the whole enchilada. To be truly charming, it takes more than saying those magic words. You need to have a great laugh, to learn to engage people with a compelling story, to be able to comment in a lively conversation without taking over, to know about current events, to have an opinion but be willing to listen to others, and to ask questions about things people are introducing you to. In short, you need to be interesting and interested.

Being charming isn't just about batting your eyelashes. It's about opening your mouth and using it wisely.

"I can do anything you want me to do, so long as I don't have to speak." —Model Linda Evangelista

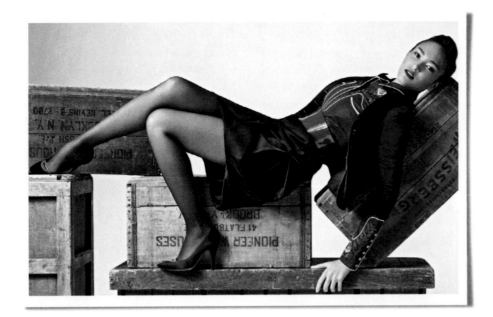

"Being a charming person is being respectful of your common man and appreciating people for who they are and what potential they possess."

—Naima Mora

THE SILENT ERA

Circa the late 1880s through the late 1920s, the first movies ever made were silent. Ordinary people became huge movie stars (alongside trained theater actors) based on the way they looked. Acting consisted of making exaggerated facial expressions and employing broad body language to express feelings and actions. To the modern eye, this style of acting seems ridiculous and downright campy.

In 1927, Al Jolson spoke the prophetic words, "Wait a minute, you ain't heard nothing yet!" Actors started to speak for the first time, and audiences could finally put a voice with a face. For the popular actors who came from theater, this wasn't an issue, as they knew how to speak. However, for many others, panic set in. No longer would wild gesticulations, the ability to make big, googly eyes, or the dubious skill of taking a cream pie in the face suffice. Now they'd need real vocal skills to charm audiences.

You may not remember her name now, but screen supernova Norma Talmadge was a megastar who was known for her sweet image on the silent screen. When she opened her mouth, however, Talmadge, who was raised in Brooklyn, had a thick accent that was completely at odds with the way the public perceived her and her movie career ended practically overnight.

Many foreigners had become famous for their exotic mystery. The world waited with bated breath to hear what Swedish actress Greta Garbo would sound like. When she finally yielded to the demand, headlines around the world broadcast GARBO SPEAKS! and the public was charmed by her accent. Hungarian-born Vilma Banky, on the other hand, had an accent so pronounced that no one could understand what she was saying. Charlie Chaplin, perhaps the first worldwide celebrity, wisely chose never to speak in his films, because he feared how American audiences would respond when they heard their icon emit a thick Cockney accent!

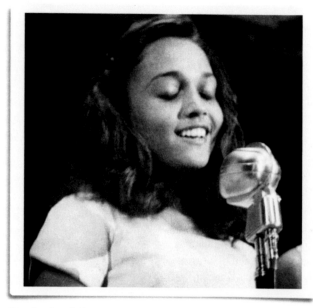

My mother, who easily charmed audiences at an early age with her beautiful singing voice

THE NEXT VOICE YOU HEAR...

Check out these entertaining classic films
that illustrate women who either learn to charm and rise to the top
by overcoming their terrible speaking voices or succumb
to their bad diction and fall to the bottom.

- **JUDY HOLLIDAY** in *Born Yesterday* (1950)
A millionaire has to hire a tutor to help his good-looking but foul-sounding girlfriend become a lady of charm and sophistication.

- **JEAN HAGEN** in *Singin' in the Rain* (1952)
A great take on the silent-to-sound era. Glamorous silent-film star Lina Lamont sounds like a cartoon mouse when she speaks, so her voice is dubbed and the public adores her . . . that is, until she has to speak before a live audience!

- **AUDREY HEPBURN** in *My Fair Lady* (1964)
A snobbish phonetics professor accepts a challenge to transform a gutter-mouthed street urchin into a presentable woman of high society.

- **JULIA ROBERTS** in *Pretty Woman* (1990)
A man falls in love with a once-vulgar prostitute after he discovers her inner charm.

- **RACHAEL LEIGH COOK** in *She's All That* (1999)
A high school jock makes a bet that he can turn an unattractive and socially inept girl into the school's prom queen.

- **QUEEN LATIFAH** in *Bringing Down the House* (2003)
A lonely man falls for a charming, brainy bombshell while chatting online. When they meet in person, she's an unrefined prison escapee and turns his life upside down.

From time to time, I've been surprised when a seemingly stunning model has stomped through a shoot, treating the makeup artists and the lighting crew like servants, and ultimately leaving me with a sour impression because of her "holier than thou" attitude. Why bother if you are not going to engage with people and enjoy what you're doing? I've come to the conclusion that the girls who pull this routine are actually very insecure. Treating my highly talented staff with an "I don't give a damn" approach while trying to seduce my lens is probably the result of being scared that they don't know how to speak or be courteous, and are unsure of their intelligence. That equates to the opposite of charm. And even a modicum of charm can make the difference. Caring about what you are doing seems like a no-brainer. Yet, some people actually believe they can get away with living life without putting any effort into it—though it's mind-boggling that they would even want to. The world owes them, and they're gonna get their due, dammit, and you're supposed to just hand it over to them, like it or not! Yeah, well, that attitude might work if you're knocking over a liquor store, but when it comes to winning friends and influencing people? Good luck, honey.

DOWNLOAD

SONGS ABOUT... WINNING AND LOSING THE ORAL ASSAULT

"What are words for when no one listens anymore?"

"Words" —MISSING PERSONS

"You Talk Too Much" —RUN DMC

"Jive Talkin'" —BEE GEES

"Really Saying Something" —BANANARAMA

"Wordy Rappinghood" —TOM TOM CLUB

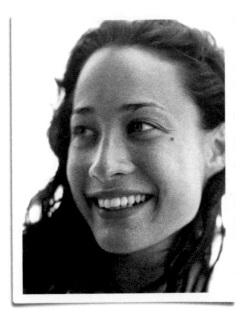

"At a casting studio in New York, there's an image in the waiting area depicting a crowd of people all staring at a leggy blonde, and these very poignant words: 'Everyone is staring at you because you are being loud and obnoxious. Please keep it down.'"
—Crissy Barker

THE ART OF CONVERSATION

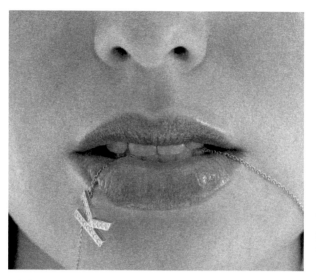

Kaiulani Swan

Being charming is not about being the loudest or funniest person in the room. Sure, someone can strike you as being charismatic or a real character, but to be truly charming is to make the person you are talking to feel special. So just as important as knowing how to be well-spoken is knowing how to listen. By listening and responding directly to what someone says, you give up on waiting to get your sound bite in. You become fully engaged in the conversation. We all know people who, the minute you see them, start rattling on about the lowdown on their life. How successful they have been, all the exciting things they have planned, and how they are almost too busy to even deal with all the attention—*yawn*! How many times have you felt invisible when a motormouth like that starts in? You could be on the phone with a person like that, put down the receiver, go to the kitchen to make yourself a sandwich, check your e-mail, and even walk the dog without the voice on the other end of the line relenting—let alone noticing.

The secret to being charming is not talking about yourself—fancy that. Talking about yourself means less work for you, because who needs to read a book, or see a movie, or read the news to blather on about their favorite subject—"and another thing about me!" By being a good listener and asking poignant questions, you can turn the spotlight away from yourself and onto the person you're talking to. And by being the kind of person who pays attention to what is going on in the world, you will likely have a wealth of references to draw on in relating to their story (versus pulling the conversation back to "Oh! Something like that happened to *me*!"). You'll leave people feeling special and charmed by their conversations with you. You don't really need to talk about yourself anyway. You know all your own stories already. And there's a bonus: By keeping your cards close to your chest, you will appear more mysterious and exciting. Leave them wanting more! How wonderful it is to be intriguing. Once you stop volunteering all your particulars every chance you get, it won't be long until they'll be asking you the questions.

THE GIFT OF GAB

I am always impressed by a great talk-show host. These people have the incredible talent of being able to sit down daily with a wide range of people, from politicians to pop stars, from athletes to authors, and have an illuminating, entertaining, and meaningful conversation. People like Oprah Winfrey, Ellen DeGeneres, and, of course, the irrepressible Tyra Banks are able to make others feel comfortable and ask just the right questions to help the audience get to know who the person really is. Guests invariably come off as interesting and walk away feeling special. How do talk-show hosts do it? Charm. They know how to win over their guests and audiences alike.

Take Heidi Klum as another example. Heidi exudes an infectious charm. If you've ever seen her interviewed, you realize that, in addition to her lovely looks, she is very intelligent, funny, and articulate. Look her up on YouTube and you can see her cracking up hosts on talk-show couches and camping it up in her "Santa Baby" Victoria's Secret commercial. Then, if you really want a laugh, search down the hard-to-find Heidi Klum's *Funny Boob Video*—her tongue-in-chic wit shines through in everything she does. It's no wonder she's had so many successes (including being nominated for multiple awards as the host of *Project Runway* and *Germany's Next Top Model*).

WHAT THE WORLD NEEDS NOW

In most walks of life, charm is in sadly short supply. We see it as unnecessary additional baggage. Then, at the end of a date, dinner with the in-laws, or a job interview, we wonder why we didn't get a second date, a return invitation, or the position we applied for.

My wife's grandfather is perhaps the most charming man I've ever met. He's debonair and modest, yet successful and rich in life. He has an ability to laugh and smile in difficult situations—and he has kind eyes. I mention this because I imagine we all know someone who has kind eyes. They look upon all with care and approval, urging you onward and upward. It's not good enough to just be saying the right thing if you're thinking the opposite, because chances are your eyes will give you away and you'll come off insincere—or worse, tedious.

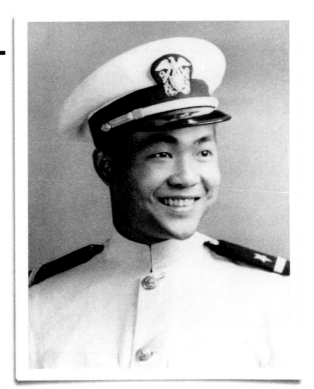

Crissy's grandfather, Jack Chin

Quick Challenge
Charm First Lady-Style

Google the words *Michelle Obama charm* and you will see a plethora of headlines about our first lady's ability to win over national leaders, former first ladies, Russian children, and even the queen of England. And not via political muscle—all via her magical charisma. Take a second to read the articles. You may just end up with a new anecdote to use when charming someone at your next soirée. Perhaps when you are complimenting someone's kind eyes.

When photographing people it's very important that I relate to them in some manner, and it's best if I can get them relaxed enough to let their guard down. In order to do that, I have to forget about whatever there might be about the person I don't care for. I'm not being booked to make a judgment call on someone, but rather to take their picture. Look, we don't always like everyone we have to work with and we all need to deal with difficult people sometimes; that's what being a professional is about. My trick is to try and be as charming as possible.

It often means biting my tongue, asking questions I don't initially think I really care to know the answers to, or "befriending" models with whom, on the surface, it seems I have nothing in common. That may sound deceptive and insincere, but it is a part of life. And you know what? More often than not, people surprise me. I find out things I never would have known

otherwise. I've learned that I can't pretend to think that my interests are more important than someone else's, nor can I let my personal feelings get in the way of doing the best job I can do.

By breaking down barriers and making my subject feel at home, I aim to lure them into a comfort zone that will allow me to succeed. I'll ask them about their family, their day, or what they're doing that weekend, but I also try to discuss the shoot concept, and ideas, and get their input and suggestions. Whether I use their ideas is not the issue; I want to make them feel that they are a part of the team and not the victim of a firing squad. The point is, if you arm yourself with charm, you have an important tool you can draw on in life's challenging moments. It'll put others at ease, and you won't walk away feeling you've done anything less than you could have done.

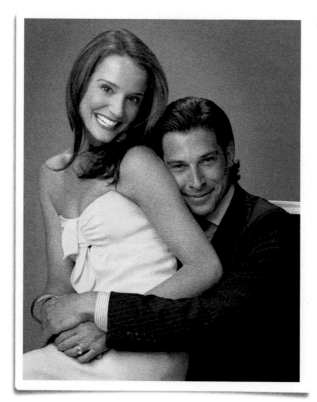

"Posing with your partner can be pretty awkward. There are a million things running through your head—how is he coming across on camera? Do I have lipstick on my teeth? Do we look too pose-y together? It can all just throw you off-balance. But when your photographer helps you feel totally sexy in your own skin, that vibe comes through so clearly in the photos. You see it in your eyes, your smile, the way you naturally pose. . . . It all comes together to create the perfect shot." — Leah Wyar, beauty director, *Cosmopolitan*, with her fiancé, Nick Romito

THE BODY LANGUAGE EQUATION

Scholars assert that nonverbal communication can account for more than 75 percent of the impact of a message. Assuming that's true, every action we make conveys what we mean and what we feel, as much or more than our words do. Of course, the significance of a body gesture can vary depending on the specifics of a situation (you might be shifting your weight because you have back trouble, not because you're bored), but here are some meanings experts agree on:

- **ARMS CROSSED ACROSS THE CHEST**
  - = disinterest
- **ARMS UNFOLDED**
  - = openness, positivity
- **HANDS ON KNEES**
  - = readiness
- **CROSSED LEGS** (unless in a skirt)
  - = lack of interest, being withdrawn
- **STANDING WITH LEGS AT SHOULDER WIDTH**
  - = being relaxed, grounded
- **STANDING WITH A VERY WIDE STANCE**
  - = power, dominance
- **STANDING TALL**
  - = confidence, health
- **SHIFTING WEIGHT FROM SIDE TO SIDE**
  - = distraction, uncomfortableness, or boredom
- **TILTING OF THE HEAD**
  - = boredom and/or confusion
- **AVERTING THE GAZE**
  - = disbelief
- **EXCESSIVE BLINKING** (or complete absence of blinking)
  - = lying
- **ECHOING AND MIRRORING**
  - = sexual interest

PUTTING YOUR MONEY WHERE YOUR UNFOLDED ARMS ARE

I've used the term *oral assault* throughout this chapter specifically because we have the ability to say one thing but communicate any number of things. All it takes is a change in our tone of voice. We all know how easy it is to send completely the wrong message. If you tell someone they have beautiful eyes, it might be meant as a compliment, but by the tone of your voice it could sound like a come-on or sarcasm. That is why being in control of your tone is so vital.

And it doesn't stop there either. Finessing your body language is just as important as controlling your tone. You don't want people to say, "She was certainly pretty to look at and she talked a good game, but she seemed uncomfortable in her own skin" any more than you want them to say, "She sounded great, but I wasn't really sure what she meant."

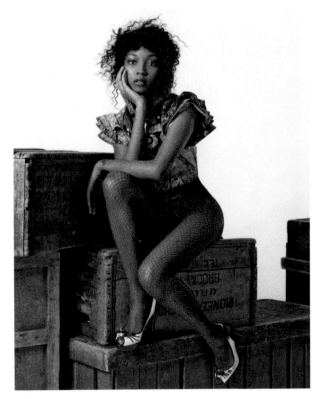

ANTM contestant Bre Skullark

When it comes to tone of voice and how it affects meaning, a case in point is Caridee English. She's become a good friend of mine, but back when we were shooting in Barcelona, she and I had a memorable little run-in. I was chatting with the girls, trying to encourage and excite them before our upcoming bullring shoot. Caridee took an unnecessary risk by cracking a joke at my expense. Personally, I wasn't actually too offended at the time, as I knew she was just joking around with me, but it did make me take pause that she would talk to one of the judges in such a disrespectful manner.

Caridee asked me whether the stick I was holding in my hand as I stood there talking was in fact the same one that was stuck in my butt at the previous judging! I guess she felt I had come down on her too hard and thought an attempt to be "cute and funny" would break the ice.

Of course, Caridee didn't really intend to be disrespectful. Had her tone come off as more aggressive than joking when she originally asked me the question, she could have offended me. But her tone saved her even when her words condemned her. And later, she saw the error of her ways and sincerely and humbly apologized. Again, saying you're sorry is one thing; sounding like you mean it is another. And here's the kicker: Her ability to convey sincerity in her apology charmed me almost more than she could have done had the incident never occurred!

Perhaps that explains why charm has been described as "deceptive"—with charm, you can win people over in the most unlikely of times.

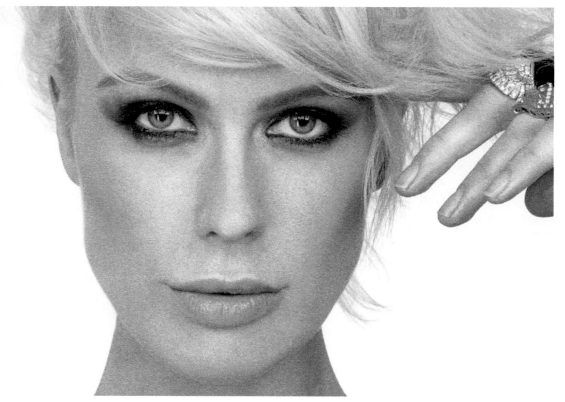

Caridee English

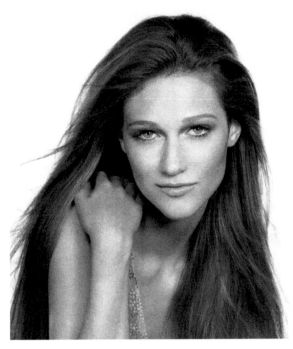

ANTM winner Nicole Fox

1. THE MANY WAYS TO SAY THINGS 🎬

Prepare your video camera and memorize this one line: "What have you been doing?"

Now you are going to repeat this line five times, but every time you say it I want the line to have a different meaning.

1. First, imagine you have just come home and found that your kid brother has made an awful mess. Putting the strength in the "What" conveys a question, in the sense of "What in the world?" You have no idea what's been going on. Stress the first word. "*What* have you been doing?"

2. Now, pretend you have just run into an old friend who was never much of a looker and who now looks absolutely amazing. It is a question of intrigue as to what her secret is. Does she have a new hairdo, has she lost weight, or is she just really happy? You want to know. Put the emphasis on the "have." "What *have* you been doing?"

3. This time it is an accusation as well as a question. Somebody's been up to no good, and you know who! It's the "you" you're addressing! You smell something rotten in Denmark, and you don't like it. So try it with the "you" getting the emphasis. "What have *you* been doing?"

4. Round four, your sister promised an hour ago to do the dishes while you ran to the market. You return to find her in front of the TV, phone in hand, finishing a box of chocolates, and the dishes in the sink piled sky-high. She didn't do what you thought she was going to do and now you want an explanation! Accent the "been." "What have *been* doing?"

5. Oh, this time you're hopping mad. The little brat next door has dug up your beautiful flowerbed and made it into a pit of mud. Feel free to yell! Put everything into the last word. "What have you been *doing*?"

When you upload these to your portfolio or simply watch them back, you'll see that you can say the same thing in many different ways. It all depends on your tone. If you had fun with this, try it again using just the word "really."

You can't believe it. *"Really?"*
There's no way. *"Really?"*
I had no idea! *"Really?"*
You've got to be kidding. *"Really?"*
This new car is free and it's yours. *"Really?!"*

2. FUNNY GIRL

Although I stand by what I've said about not having to be the loudest or funniest in the room to command it, I do think people are going to see your charm better when you are "on." You want your energy to show, and you want people to know you're ready to laugh. Google "comic monologues for women." Then just pick one at random and print it out.

In front of your video camera, try reading just a line or two from the monologue. If you are digging it, try the whole thing. No need to memorize. Just practice your diction, sounding clear and enunciating words properly. When you're feeling good about the flow, turn the camera on. Try to dazzle. Play up the humor. Do a few takes. Pick your favorite and upload it to your portfolio or save it to your desktop.

Watching it back, how would you rate your charm level? Think in the third person. Are you happy with the person you're watching? Does she engage with you? Is she fun? Do you like her tone? How's her body language? If you see room for improvement, try it again. We're in no hurry, and we want you to sparkle.

3. SPOKESPERSONA

No doubt you've seen modeling-competition challenges on TV where the contestants have to do a commercial? They're getting to the point when their Beauty Equation should start to come through strong and clear, the point when a girl's charm might be the single thing that determines whether she's a finalist.

Pick any item you have nearby: a book or CD you love, your favorite item from your makeup drawer, or a new top that looks great on you. Think about a few lines you could say about your product to show the audience how fantastic it is. Set up your video camera and shoot a little commercial.

When you upload it or save it, watch it back and ask yourself, did your charm help sell your product or is the poor product going to have to sell itself?

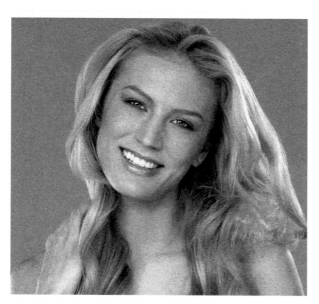

IT'S important to believe in what you're saying. Commitment and faith in what you do can easily be disbelieved if, when you describe what you're doing, you sound unsure of yourself. The words you use are important, but you also need to think about what the rest of you is saying. Always be aware of your vocal approach and body language, especially when meeting someone for the first time. Avoid being negative, but also don't become a bullshit merchant in order to please. There is good to be found in almost anything—seek it out and verbalize it!

Shannon Rusbuldt, twenty-three, model, capturing charm

159

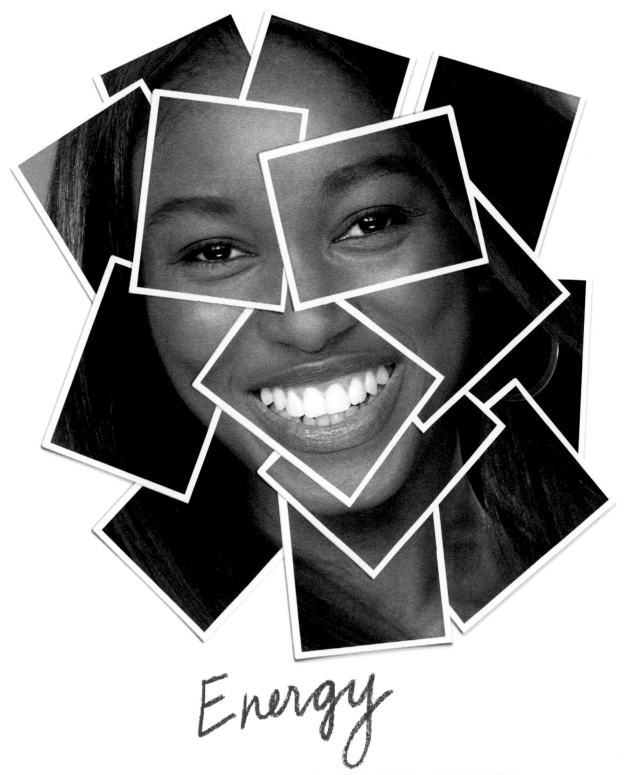

Energy

TO VITALIZE YOUR BEAUTY THROUGH AMBITION

> "The energy of the mind is the essence of life."
>
> —**Aristotle**

Pump Up the Jam: *the teach*

THE BIG BANG

Ever since the dawn of time, the universe has relied mightily on one thing—the thing that makes life move forward, the thing that gets us out of bed every morning, and the thing that continues to build cities and nations. What is it? Energy, of course! Every movement, thought, and gesture is the result of that energy, whether it be the electricity that runs through power lines or the impulse that's sent from your brain to your lips when you smile. There is energy all around us. Sometimes you can see it, but most of the time you can't. Yet there it is, always pushing ahead, ensuring that our world doesn't come to a grinding halt.

Scientists are on a never-ending quest to harness energy. They try to capture it and dissect its elements in an attempt to truly understand just what it is and how it can be used. One of the greatest minds in the history of Western civilization devoted himself to understanding the meaning of energy and sharing his findings with the rest of us. Who was it? Albert Einstein, of course!

$$E = mc^2$$

I'm sure you recognize this. It is perhaps the world's most famous and recognizable equation. Introduced in 1905, Einstein's formula is now commonly referred to as the special theory of relativity. Broken down, it is saying that energy converts to matter at the speed of light squared. Huh?

Think that sounds complicated, try this: In physics, "mass–energy equivalence" is the concept that the mass of a body is a measure of its energy content. The mass of a body as measured on a scale is always equal to the total energy inside, divided by a constant (c^2), which changes the units appropriately where E is energy, m is mass, and c is the speed of light in a vacuum. Whew! I'm exhausted just trying to wrap my head around it.

What does it all mean? Basically, it means a small amount of matter can release a huge amount of energy. In the scope of the universe, each of us, compared to the massiveness of, say, the sun, represents a pretty small amount of matter, but the energy we are capable of releasing through what we say and what we do is huge!

The theory has been used to help explain how a nuclear bomb works. And a hundred years later, it was co-opted by Mariah Carey for her album title $E=MC^2$, only her formula was "(E) Emancipation (=) of (MC) Mariah Carey (2) to the second power." Fierce, but not very scientific!

As for me, when I was back in England in sixth form (the equivalent of senior year in the States), a seventeen-year-old science buff, I was completely and utterly fascinated by Einstein's theory and remember having my own big-bang moment. It was as if the universe were being created for the first time, and of course, it was—my universe, that is. In trying to relate the theory back to my own life, I concluded that the "energy" was what was required to do anything and get anywhere, and all I had to do was to harness it. I also took into consideration that if energy simply exists—that is, it cannot be created or destroyed—it was going to be up to me to find it in myself—the "mass"—and utilize it. I took the "speed" to mean that I should waste no time. I essentially motivated myself to grab life by the horns, and I shook my whole world up like a soda bottle. I've been waiting for the bubbles to die down ever since.

THAT'S REALLY GETTING IT TOGETHER!

One of the most attractive elements of any Beauty Equation is energy. Motivated people draw others to them with the fact that they seem to want to be a part of life and make things happen. Ambition drives this motivation and helps people make their dreams come true and reach the highest peaks.

I've seen girls come down the runway who seemingly don't know why they're there. I look at them and wonder how they managed to get a booking so many other girls are dying to have when they don't even seem motivated to be there. Did someone tell them, "You should be a model," and then they just lucked into it? When there are no answers to the questions about their motives, I can only assume there is no ambition deep inside. It's just an arbitrary choice in an uninspired life.

Self-determination is the key to inspiring us to make choices of our own free will, hopefully driven by natural human motivation. When you decide you should pursue something based on what other people have said or because things in the outside world are interfering with your intuition, you are going to end up with a big fizzle of negative energy at the end of the rainbow, not a pot of gold. Doing things others want you to do is fueling their ambitions, not your own. I often encounter "stage mothers" who are pushing their daughters into a modeling career, most likely because it was a

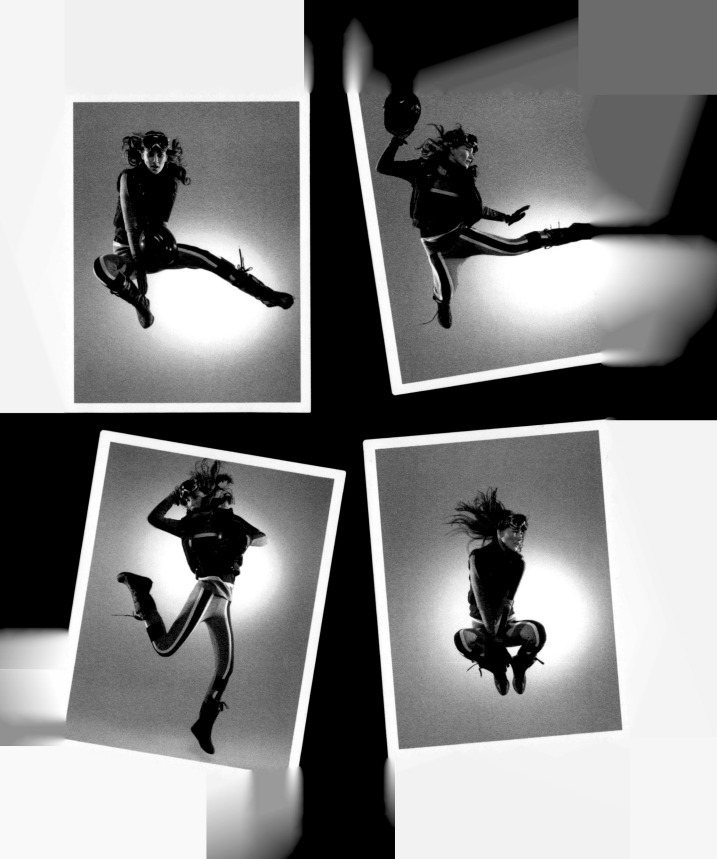

dream they never fulfilled when they had their chance. It is very difficult to go after what you really want when you have a parent breathing down your neck, telling you what you should want. In the words of Stephen R. Covey, who wrote the best-selling book *The Seven Habits of Highly Effective People*, "Motivation is a fire from within. If someone else tries to light that fire under you, chances are it will burn very briefly." Well said.

On the other hand, when I meet a girl on the show—or anyone anywhere—driven with energy, ambition, and motivation, I am always impressed. It's admirable when people know who they are and where they are going. When you ask a question, they give you a clear answer—not this "Oh, like, um, maybe? I don't know. . . . Hadn't really thought about it before." How can you exist in a world as vast and exciting as ours and not ponder what you want out of life? Sadly, I fear many people don't. But for those who do, life can produce some rather extraordinary rewards, including beauty and a long and fascinating journey.

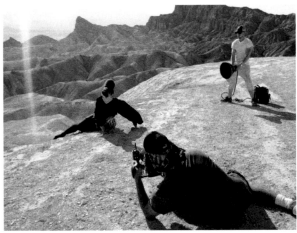
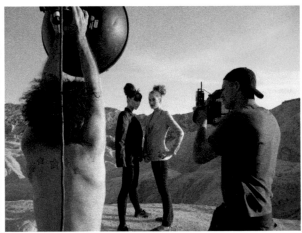
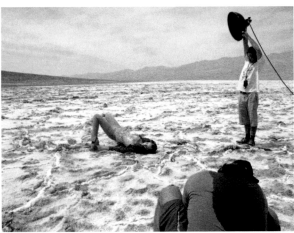
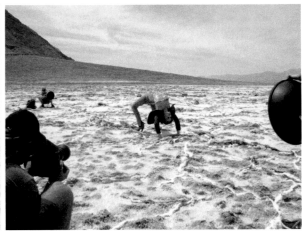

This grueling shoot in Death Valley epitomizes energy. Models Stephanie Wood and Ruby Corley, working in 110-degree weather, are rolling around on razor-sharp crystals determined to get the shot. Hard work always pays off.

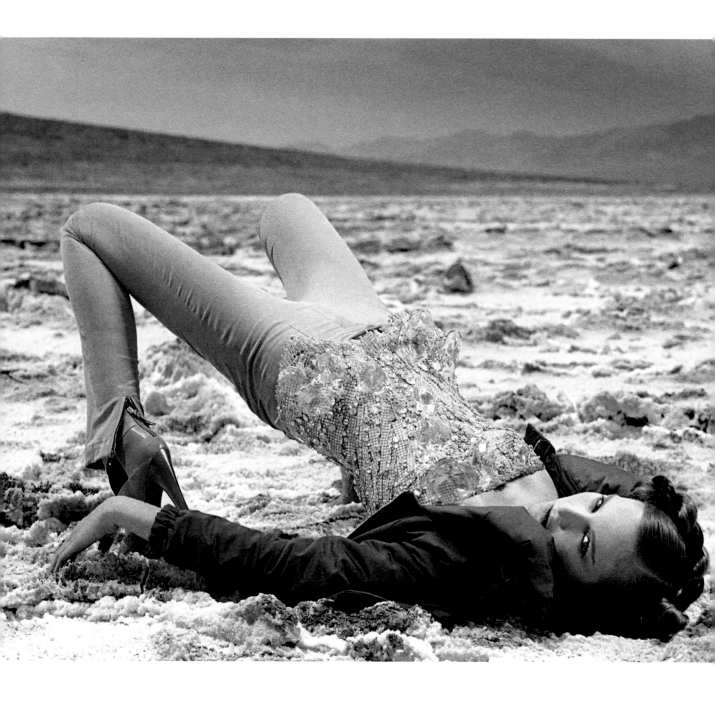

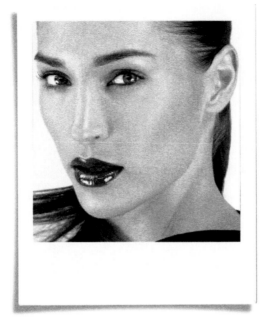

ANN AWAY WE GO

ANN MARKLEY

"Ralph Waldo Emerson once said, 'There is a guidance in each of us, and by lowly listening we shall hear the right word.' I came to find my own inner beauty by quieting my mind and really listening to myself . . . really listening to the things that were inside of me. Those are the things that give me my inner beauty."

When I first met Ann, she exhibited energy in a number of obvious ways. First, she is an athlete. She played water polo for the National Collegiate Athletic Association and has the figure to prove it. Second, she is exceptionally bright and had been working as a pharmacy technician to put herself through college. But little did I know then the true depths of her energy.

Ann clearly has the ambition to dive into any competition. When she feels she has a lot to learn, she has the gusto to go for it. Early on, she found herself criticized for not using her eyes to their fullest advantage. But her passion would not be squelched. She's the kind of person who, when confronted with constructive criticism, pulls herself up and tries even harder. Her energy leads her to self-motivate.

Ann's ambition continues on and her motivation for success drives her. You know that moment on reality shows where the teary-eyed departing contestant says, "You haven't seen the last of me"? Well, Ann meant it. She moved to New York and has become solidly successful in the real-world business of modeling. By following her heart, she's gone on to grace magazine covers; do commercial work for Target, L'Oreal, and Ray-Ban; and walk the runway both here and abroad for the likes of Marc Bouwer, Cynthia Rowley, and Nicole Miller. Oh, and she and Naima Mora were the trophy girls for the *Fifty-seventh Annual Primetime Emmy Awards.* Not bad. Not bad at all.

Says Ann, "I think the best advice that I could give would be for girls to just be who they are. Work on the inner beauty first and the outer beauty will fall into place. I certainly didn't consider myself to be a beautiful woman until I was happy with who I was on the inside."

"How the hell can a person go to work in the morning and come home in the evening and have nothing to say?"

—Singer/songwriter John Prine,
from his frequently rerecorded song
"Angel from Montgomery"

DOWNLOAD

SONGS ABOUT ENERGY . . .
THAT ARE LOADED WITH DYNAMITE!

"Everyone knows an ant can't move a rubber tree plant . . . but he's got high hopes!"

....

"High Hopes" —FRANK SINATRA

"I'm So Excited" —THE POINTER SISTERS

"Celebration" —KOOL & THE GANG

"Exceptional" —JOJO

"Breakaway" —KELLY CLARKSON

"Pump Up the Jam" —TECHNOTRONIC

What excites you? What are you passionate about? What is it that you desire from life? These questions are the keys that open the floodgates of energy. And you are your own locksmith. Only you can open the doors of your mind to explore your own awe and mystery. When you take the time to open these doors, your own big bang comes about. First you begin to see what you want, then a spontaneous combustion occurs that will produce enough energy to get you where you need to go.

Energy is exciting! Think about those physical displays of energy that are so awesome to behold—like Old Faithful in Yellowstone National Park when it erupts. It's a thrilling sight that really lets you know that energy exists. Or think about Las Vegas, where all the power of electricity generated at the Hoover Dam gets channeled into igniting the gazillions of multicolored lightbulbs on the Strip that are burning so bright that it turns the night sky into the brightest day. Exhilarating. Or think about Bruce Springsteen in concert. Love or hate his music, he is so alive onstage that he practically bursts at the seams with energy. How do you think the Boss does it, concert after concert, year after year? Having sold more than 61 million records in the United States alone, he certainly doesn't do it because he has to. And he's not drinking Red Bull all day to create the illusion that he is electric. He is finding his own Beauty Equation through desire and motivation—a desire to please an audience with his music, and the motivation to get it all together and get the job done—and have a great time while he's at it. Energy is fun!

Betsey Johnson is full of energy. I photographed her for her sixtieth birthday for *Paper* magazine.
She danced and cartwheeled all around my studio. You'd have thought it was her sixteenth!

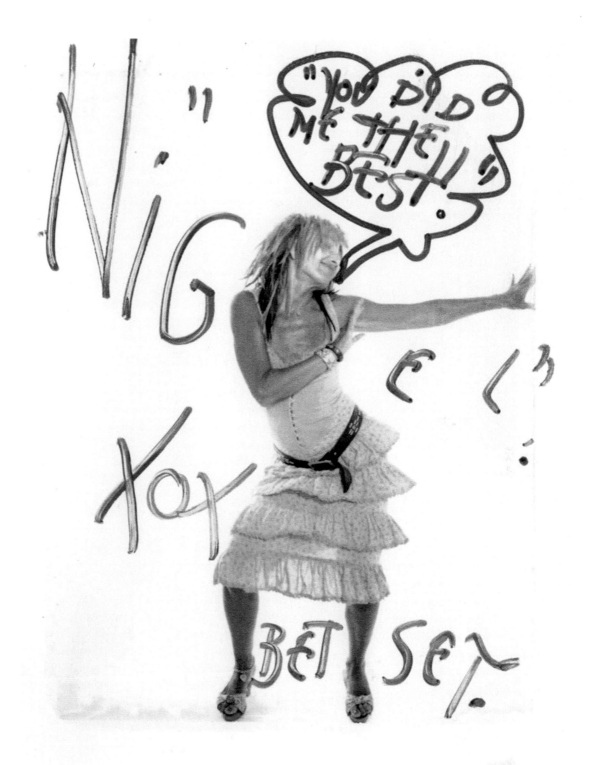

Life is a funny thing. Sometimes your ambitions manifest in ways you never imagined possible. And no matter how much energy, ambition, and motivation you might have, it's not always easy. Everyone's journey is going to be filled with ups and downs. Mine certainly has been.

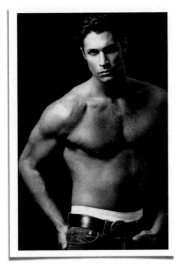

In my earlier modeling days

When I was eighteen and, as I've mentioned, decided to try my hand at modeling, my parents were none too keen on the idea of my taking a year off before starting school to see what this newly inspired passion had in store for me. It wasn't easy to convince my folks that I would be entirely self-sufficient and would even take a night job should I need any supplementary income. They finally agreed, though, and taking a calculated risk, I embarked on the biggest and most exciting adventure of my life.

It wasn't long before I got a booking for a modeling job in Milan, Italy. The client was paying for my flight, hotel, and food, plus providing me a nice fee. It seemed like things were really coming together. Armed with little more than an overnight bag and about fifty bucks, I headed to the airport, filled with excitement and anticipation. However, the universe is very mysterious.

You've heard of Murphy's law, of course. "Anything that can go wrong will go wrong"? The traffic on the way to the airport was horrific, bumper-to-bumper hell. At one point, my taxi was stuck in this half-mile tunnel that leads to Heathrow Airport. Talk about time moving at the speed of light—the hands on my watch seemed to be spinning forward. The sweat was pouring down my temples and the possibility of my missing the flight to my first big booking was quickly looking more like a reality. Panic!

On seeing the light at the end of the tunnel—literally—I grabbed my bag, paid my hapless driver, and ran for my life. I ran into the terminal, gasping for air. I made a mad dash for the gate. It was then I learned my flight had been delayed. Of course, I was greatly relieved, but I was also exhausted.

Finally arriving in Milan, I went straight to the hotel on my call sheet. But there seemed to be a slight problem. The hotel had no record of my reservation and was fully booked. Bloody hell. I didn't have a credit card or enough cash to pay up front for a room—anywhere! I tried calling my agent, but of course it was Sunday, and he wasn't at the office. I instinctually started dialing my parents' number. Who else do you call when you find yourself in a jam? *But wait!* I suddenly remembered the promise I had made. I was my own master now, and this was my trip. I had to think on my feet.

Bag in hand and a few pound notes in my pocket, I headed into the center of town. There is a large castle near the main train station. It has a lovely garden—and a plethora of park benches. Now, I can't recommend this to anyone, nor would I ever want my children to follow in these particular footsteps, but it was sink or swim. So, believe it or not, I started my modeling career after spending the night on a park bench! Not very glamorous, but I felt it was my only option and I was determined to turn this opportunity into a success.

Fortunately, I got through what could have been a very dangerous situation unscathed. I was emboldened by sheer determination to battle through the situation without asking for help. That night will

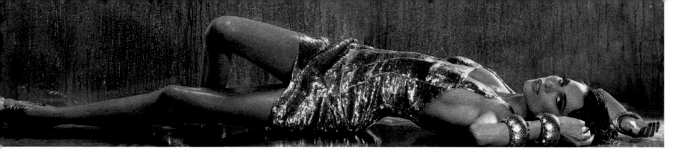

Alina Puscau, slipping and nearly injuring her arm on a very wet set of a photo shoot for *Tatler* magazine (the consummate professional, she turned the fall into a genius shot)

always be a benchmark in my life (bad pun intended). I did some serious growing up on that bench and felt more confident about what I was capable of overcoming than I ever could have if I had been flown in on a private jet and spent the night in a five-star hotel. In the morning, I washed up in the train station and went directly to my job, as if nothing had happened. The shoot was a success. As you can well imagine, though, I was all the more delighted to check into my hotel the following night!

The moral of my adventure is certainly not that you should go out and spend the night on a park bench, but that sometimes life gives you lemons and you have to have the motivation and energy to turn them into lemonade.

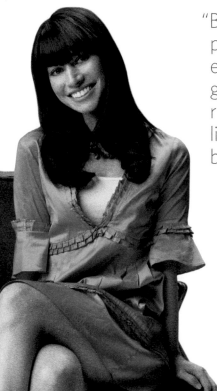

"Beauty is a positive, warm energy that gives you a radiant glow like no blush or bronzer can do."

—Beauty and fashion expert Rebekah George

Quick Challenge
Name That Mantra

Originating in ancient India, a mantra is a sound, word, or group of words that you speak to yourself, either out loud or in your head, over and over again. Through repetition, some believe, a mantra is capable of bringing about transformation.

Remember the story from childhood, *The Little Engine That Could*? It was about an optimistic and hard-working little train that accepts a seemingly impossible challenge but overcomes the odds by chanting the mantra, "I think I can; I think I can; I think I can."

Think of a saying that helps motivate you, one you can call on whenever you need a little push. What kinds of words focus your eyes on the prize? It doesn't need to be original. It can be as cornball as that saying from the poster of the kitten hanging on to a tree branch for dear life, "Hang in there, baby." It can be as simple as "Go for it," "Just do it," or "Make it work." If you are at a loss for mantras, here are some additional classics to get your juices flowing:

"Life's too short!"
"Let's get this party started!"
"Onward and upward!"
"Breathe."
"No worries!"
"Love what you do; do what you love."
"Done is better than perfect."
"When it's right, it's right!"
"It is what it is."
"One step at a time."
"*C'est la vie!*"
"Let's go!"
"Om shanti om."

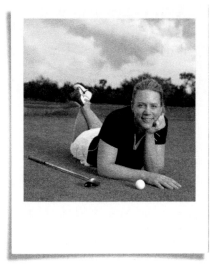

Annika Sörenstam in a Make-A-Wish Foundation ad campaign

HOW TO SWING IT

ANNIKA SÖRENSTAM

In the world of professional golf, Annika Sörenstam is a legend. When she first picked up a golf club at age twelve, already accomplished in tennis, soccer, and skiing, little did she know she had also picked up her ticket to international success. Today Annika is one of the most victorious golfers in the sport's history and only the second woman ever to play on the male-dominated PGA tour.

Like most smart athletes (and models), she knew that she wouldn't stay at the top of her game forever. Before stepping away from competitive golf in 2008, she had already begun to develop other interests, and today she has transitioned into a supersuccessful entrepreneur, businesswoman, and philanthropist. Combining her major passions—golf, fitness, and charitable works—Annika has ventured into various businesses under the ANNIKA banner, with the brand statement, "Share My Passion." She now has her own golf academy, charitable foundation, clothing line, and signature perfume scent. She even designs golf courses! When she closed the door on one brilliant career, she opened dozens of others and I'm sure she will be expanding on her many other talents for years to come. Annika is a stellar example of how the energy of a single person can yield a towering tidal wave of achievement.

CALL TO ACTION

> "Success is where preparation and opportunity meet."
> —Race car driver Bobby Unser

Since that night in Milan, one of my own mantras has been, "Action speaks louder than words." Having the motivation to find the energy to act is where you have to begin.

It's not that you need to know exactly what you want to do or where you are heading. I certainly didn't start with a plan. It's rather that you need to believe you are worth it—worth the motivation. Use that motivation to discover who you are, and what you want and need. With that knowledge, you'll uncover the driving force for pursuing your ambitions, one step at a time. In order to stay motivated, you need to find inspiration, so listen to your theme song or hit the gym every morning—whatever works for you.

Be prepared for change. You know that I became a photographer after modeling, but did you know that I have always loved taking photographs? Although I spent the first few years of my career in fashion as a model, I was always taking pictures, honing my eye. You never know what life has in store for you, or which of your interests or passions will end up being the thing you do for a living. Or for a second career. What a wonderful thing though, when your avocation—the thing you love to do—becomes your vocation—your paycheck.

When my modeling career started to take off in the late eighties, male models were tall and muscular, healthy and athletic. I would do shoots and walk runways with guys like Marcus Schenkenberg, Mark Vanderloo, and Paul Sculfor. The women who were in vogue at the time were Naomi Campbell, Claudia Schiffer, and Christy Turlington—curvaceous Glamourzonians. But the tides were turning. Bands like Hole, Pearl Jam, and Nirvana were invading the radio airwaves and an entirely new aesthetic was coming into vogue. Soon the previous decade's obsession with a healthy and sexy image would be replaced with a new obsession, heroin chic.

I knew I didn't have the look or physique to work this latest trend, nor did I let it bother me. Instead, I took it as the perfect opportunity to migrate to the other side of the camera on a more permanent basis. But that didn't just happen overnight. I was prepared for change. Focus is important, but having ambition and motivation doesn't mean shutting everything else out in pursuit of one goal.

SWITCHING SIDES

Getting started as a photographer was no walk in the park. To be commercially successful and make a name for yourself in any major city is no easy feat. Still, I knew I had certain advantages, as I had been working in the fashion industry for almost eight years. I had built up a good knowledge of how things worked and what people were looking for.

I worked on building my portfolio, asking fellow models and friends to pose for me. Then I asked a stunning young model named Cristen Chin, who now goes by the name Cristen Barker, to be one of my subjects. Suddenly I couldn't put my camera down. I was driven to develop my abilities, and was on the fast track to creating more exciting pictures. When that lightbulb goes off inside your head, you discover the passion within yourself. Was I looking for this? Maybe not consciously, but certainly it was brewing in my soul.

It was fate that I would meet my muse early in my career, and that she would create the energy in me to become (as Tyra so lovingly calls me on every show) a "noted fashion photographer." The more time I spent with Crissy, the more I saw her in every kind of light, every kind of mood. The more time I spent with my muse, the more my vision as a photographer would develop.

Then, in the late eighties, Mickey Boardman of *Paper* magazine asked me to shoot a spread about "male vanity," representing the shift in the male aesthetic that I had become a "victim" of. How apropos! Thrilled for the opportunity, I had an energy burst that delivered what I believed was a dynamic, artistic, and exciting set of photographs. The pictures caught

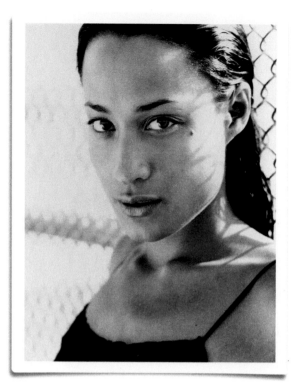

A simple test shot of Crissy when I first met her

the eyes of the tastemakers of the New York fashion world, and my new career was off and running.

Since it wasn't my first time at the rodeo, I quickly realized that the most successful and respected people among those I had the privilege of working with were those doing things the way they wanted to, whether they were hated or loved—the cardinal rule was not to be ignored. So I went for it. I found a cool loft space in the then-sordid Meatpacking District of Manhattan. What is now my studio used to be an inn of ill repute. Yep, I work in a former brothel! Once equipped with thirty small rooms where who knows what went on, the joint had been gutted and turned it into one big room. I made a few changes of my own and voilà! My very own photo studio was now open for business. What do you know? The kid who was going to be a doctor had become a New York City fashion photographer by way of being a working model. Who'da thunk it?

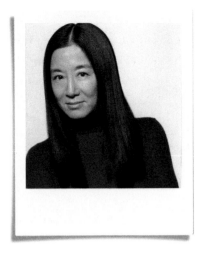

PROFILE IN ENERGY

VERA WANG

Watch the red-carpet coverage of any major awards show. How many times, when asked, "And what are you wearing?" does the glamorous star reply, "Vera Wang!" In the *Sex and the City* movie, too, the Carrie Bradshaw character models a Vera Wang wedding dress for *Vogue*. Vera is one of the top designers in the industry, and her wedding dresses are highly sought after. Well, she was one of my first commissions. I got hired to shoot a portrait of her.

Talk about a force of nature. Vera competed in the U.S. Figure Skating Championships as a teenager, earned a degree in art history from Sarah Lawrence, was a senior fashion editor for *Vogue* for sixteen years, and worked as Ralph Lauren's design director before she opened her own salon in 1990. Says Vera, "All those years of skating have carried over. I can't design anything without thinking of how a woman's body will look and move when she's wearing it."

Vera is a very big personality, a swirling ball of colorful energy, so when I first met her I was a bit intimidated. But I was also very honored that she was a fan of *mine* and had sought me out to take her picture. She knew exactly how she wanted to appear—how her hair was to be done, how her makeup should look—and she knew the feeling she wanted to exude. I listened, and apparently was able to capture what she wanted. I figured I had done something right when she bought out all rights to the photos in perpetuity. If you ever come across her bestselling book *On Weddings*, flip it over and you'll see Vera's author portrait (by Nigel Barker!).

BEATING THE ODDS

Most of my friends thought I was out of my mind to sink all my savings into a photo studio and new career. But I had my foot in the door, believed I had talent, and once again embarked on a calculated risk that in the end would pay off. I loved having a big studio space and wanted to have my own "factory" environment, like Andy Warhol. I wanted the place to be filled with activity, friends, dogs, kids, clients, creativity, and good times. In other words, *energy*!

Have you ever heard the saying, "Fake it till you make it"? Although I don't advocate trying to "fake" anything, my motivation to have such a space did create business almost out of thin air. Many of the early clients who booked me for various jobs just assumed I was hot stuff because I had this enormous studio that was buzzing with action. It gave me a lot of latitude, but it also meant that, behind the scenes, Crissy and I were scrambling to make ends meet. We worked seven-day weeks for twelve hours a day to be able to make the rent. We did everything we could to carve out a niche for ourselves in a highly competitive business. That energy to work hard and desire to get ahead was possible because we motivated each other and found inspiration in the people around us. And we pumped up the jam every morning with our own theme song: "New York, New York," by Frank Sinatra—"If I can make it there, I'll make it anywhere."

As a photographer today, I am drawn to and most enjoy shooting people who share that get-up-and-go. It's innately appealing. That sense of direction—even when the subject's end goal isn't yet clearly defined—makes me (and my lens) want to follow. The desire to try something new, take a calculated risk, and improve your performance by learning from your mistakes gives you the kind of *joie de vivre* that makes you exciting to be around.

"There are so many dancers who are too shy to speak or sing. For my first Broadway show, I was hired as a dancer, but I got to be the understudy for the lead by saying yes, I could sing and yes, I could act. I took voice lessons twice a week for six months!"

—Debbie Allen

By the turn of the twenty-first century, my career as a photographer was going quite well. I had been working with a stylist and fashion editor named Nolé Marin, who told me a new reality series called *America's Next Top Model* was looking for photographers to appear on the show and shoot challenges. Well, impressed by Tyra's transition to television producer and naturally interested in the subject matter, I had already been watching the fledgling show and was a huge fan.

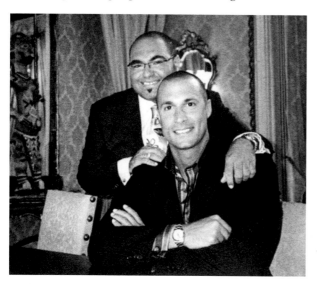

With Nolé Marin

Feeling that familiar push of ambition, I agreed to audition. It turned out to be in creative director Jay Manuel's apartment, in front of the show's executive producer at the time, the charming Anthony Dominici. Little did I know then that I'd end up friends for life with both men. When they told me later that I was hired, they also wanted to know if I'd like a more permanent role on the show—as a judge! Well, shiver me timbers and blow me down!

I knew I was gambling on another calculated risk, but I put all my chips on the table and went for it. Let's be clear: I do mean to characterize this particular life choice as a gamble. At the time, the fashion industry found TV quite gauche, and tastemakers in the industry loudly and publicly frowned on the "commercialization of the art form." Nevertheless, the idea of beaming into millions of living rooms during prime time every week potentially meant that I could take my photography to new levels, beyond what fashion currently allowed.

Today, one of the things I love about working on *ANTM* is that the shoots always feel like real jobs, not just some TV simulation. I think the fact that Tyra casts people who actually work in the fashion industry has enabled the show to be believable, where other "reality" shows have failed for their lack of reality.

I have to stop here and acknowledge the mysterious nature of the universe once more. My whole foray into the fashion world was the result of being chosen as a runner-up on a TV modeling competition. Now here I am, shoe on the other foot, having been given an opportunity to do something for which I was so uniquely qualified! Maybe that'll serve to silence the critics who say you can never become successful from competing on a reality show.

1. THE GOALPOST

Think about what your goals are in life. Maybe there's been one bursting desire inside of you for a while or several things you have been thinking about and wanting to explore. Add these to your portfolio.

Now, let's think about your goals. Are they realistic? Are they attainable? Are they in your control? It's perfectly acceptable to aim for the stars, but does your ambition and motivation match what you want to reach?

For instance, say your goal is to be rich. Is being rich a means to an end or the end to a means? Being rich is usually the result of hard work, not the outcome of a desire. You usually have to do something and do it well to end up with a big bank account. Sure, you can win the lottery, but your chances of that are less likely than being struck by lightning. Ask yourself, is it a calculated risk to take a one in 15 million chance, or is that just wishing on a star?

Analyze your goals and decide if they will take a week or a year or a decade to accomplish. Hone down your goals if they are too general. If your goal was to get in shape, make a more specific commitment to yourself, like promising to work out three days a week. All the answers are there if you know the questions to ask.

2. THE SCOREBOARD

You are going to create a vision board—a tool that allows you to visualize your energy, dreams, and ambitions, through images that represent your goals. Search the Web for the things you want to have. Look for pictures of people who inspire you. They may already be on your computer. A family member, teacher, friend, or a loyal cat might inspire you! Find photos of places you want to go or challenging adventures you'd like to tackle.

Have fun organizing and moving the images around on your vision board. When all these things are in front of you, you might discover what is most attractive and move it to the center or the top. Once you are happy with your collage and feel confident it represents the untapped potential inside you, start seeing yourself in there. Insert some of your favorite photos of yourself, maybe from our previous photo challenges. Let these images motivate you to seize the moment and start working toward your winning score in life!

3. THE END GOAL

Using your vision board as inspiration, close your eyes and project yourself into the future. Feel your passion for life, and imagine for a moment you are where you want to be in a year or two or ten. Now embrace your energy and take a self-portrait.

Add this to your portfolio and take a look at all that you can be! You can do anything you want in life, so don't waste a moment. Get out there and kick some ass!

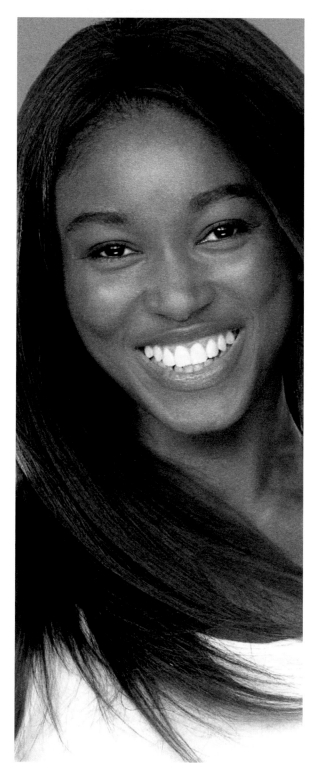

I'VE shared my own path to success as a photographer with you here in the hopes that it will inspire you to say yes to life's challenges. Do you have the energy it takes to achieve your dreams? The only way you'll ever know is to try. Whether it comes quickly or takes a lifetime, remember, it's the journey that really matters; once the chase is over, the excitement wanes. The secret is to constantly challenge yourself, knowing that by being open to change, you will meet and be forced to interact with people more educated and more developed than yourself, who perhaps even have more poise and a stronger sense of their own beauty. Accept that challenge! Aspire to have what they have. Their success doesn't mean that you are not beautiful and don't have anything to offer—your experiences are always uniquely your own. Take pride in who you are. Be willing to ruffle some feathers, don't take no for an answer (within reason), and always strive to be the best you. Trying to live life with as few regrets as possible should be motivation enough. You can't win the game of life if you don't play.

Ruwaida Jawando, twenty-three, student, capturing energy

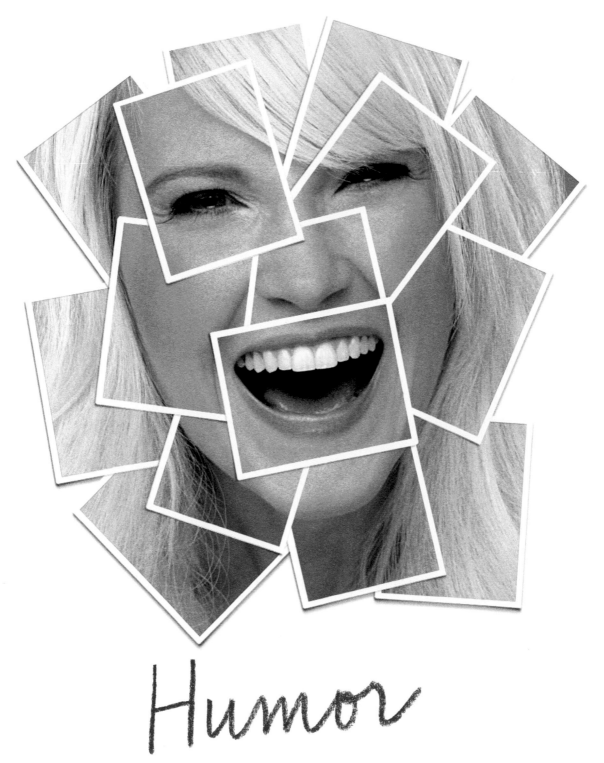

Humor

TO EMBRACE THE POWER OF WIT AND REPARTEE

> "Through humor, you can soften some of the worst blows that life delivers. And once you find laughter, no matter how painful your situation might be, you can survive it."
>
> —**Bill Cosby**

Comedy Hour: *the teach*

LADIES AND GENTLEMEN, MR. NIGEL BARKER!

"Good evening, ladies and germs. I just flew in from London and, boy, are my arms tired!" *Bada boom!* "Hard work never killed anybody, but why take a chance?" *High-hat crash.* "If truth is beauty, how come there's no Nobel Prize for makeup?" *Bada boom, crash!* "Take my wife, please! . . . Thank you, I'm here all week!" *Applause!*

Forgive my stale attempt at stand-up, but I'm making a point here. When I talk about humor, I'm not talking about the art of comedy. Comedy represents a whole universe unto itself. Jokes are carefully scripted, workshopped, and audience-tested before comics dare to share them with the world. And thank God these funny people exist, because they do keep the world laughing.

But seriously, folks, as we near the final summation of the Beauty Equation we get to one of the most important elements of them all. Take all the other elements of the equation and divide them with humor! Laughter takes the edge off nearly any difficulty and adds the final luster to your personal Beauty Equation.

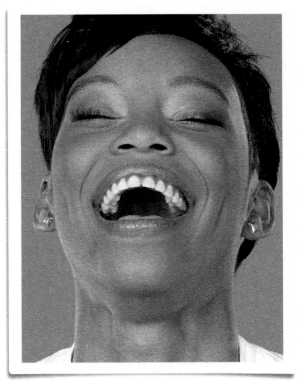

Lulu Braithwaite

CRACKIN' UP

Nothing feels better than a good chortle or guffaw! Having a sense of humor is rooted in the ability to laugh, not necessarily the ability to be funny. Of course, being funny is a great gift too. Actor and funny girl Drew Barrymore said it well (in her endorsement for *The Week* magazine): "To be smart, funny, and globally aware is a turn-on for me." That's a triple threat that is a winner in any Beauty Equation. The naturally hilarious Drew is intuitively aware of what makes a good foundation for quick wit and a sparkling repartee. Knowledge and vocabulary are excellent tools in crafting a good quip. The same tools allow you to laugh at the appropriate moment.

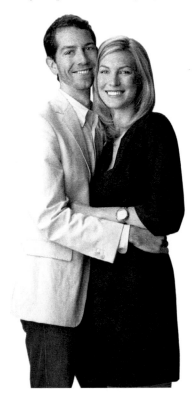

"The most beautiful women have a sense of humor. Life is too short to not spend it laughing, even at yourself!" —Janna Johnson, beauty and fitness assistant, *Elle* magazine, with boyfriend, Clayton O'Toole

Veronica Webb from our Fashion Targets Breast Cancer shoot revealing her fabulous smile

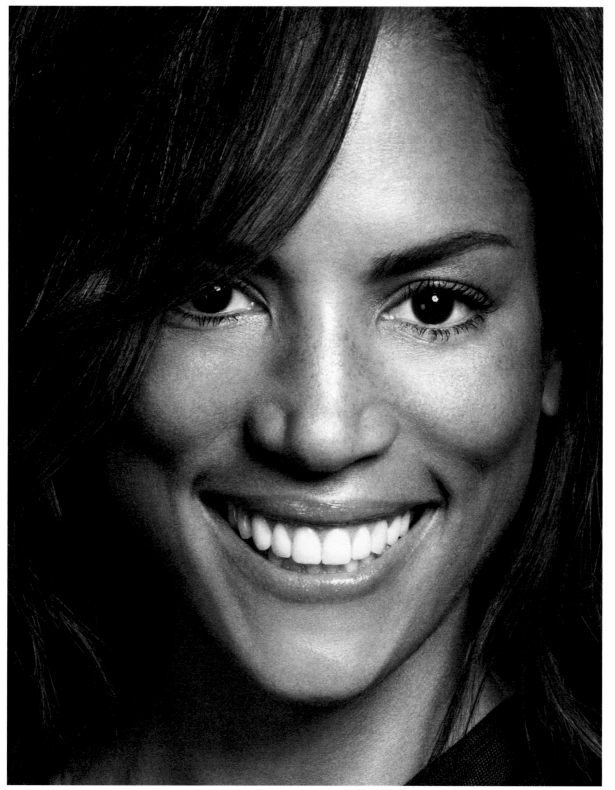

IMPROVE YOUR HUMOR QUOTIENT

Here are five sources that'll help make you a funnier person and teach you more about the world to boot:

1. **THE ONION**—Self-billed as "America's Finest News Source," this online and print periodical lampoons everyone from sports celebrities to world leaders, while serving as a primer to what's going on in the world.

2. **THE DAILY SHOW WITH JON STEWART** (and "the Best F#@king News Team Ever")—Stewart takes on current events with a slant toward the ridiculous. As long as the joke at their expense is funny, no one is safe on either side of the political aisle. Watch, and learn what the headlines are actually trying to say—or avoid saying.

3. **GOOGLE**—From Oscar Wilde to Dorothy Parker to David Letterman, great minds throughout history have developed the art of the one-liner, and thanks to the "Interwebs," their quotes are everywhere. All you have to do is run a search online! Try the combos *witty quips, funny one-liners,* or *humorous quotes.*

4. **THE WEEK**—Who has time to read every magazine and newspaper in the world? But then again, who needs to when you have this wise and witty compilation of hot topics culled from top media sources the world over? Sometimes straight, sometimes funny, this is the fast track to having the first clue about what in the blazes people are talking about.

5. **YOUR POISON OF CHOICE**—Most of us run in a certain circle of people according to our line of work (entertainment, law, fashion, health, retail, sanitation), and to make people laugh or be able to get the joke, it pays to know your business inside and out. Read something, watch something, or attend some event about "your" world, exposing yourself to something new at least once a week, and I guarantee you'll have something witty to say—eventually!

Possessing a sense of humor can mean the difference between feeling offended and feeling complimented by someone's words. What's your first reaction when someone you don't know tells you, out of the blue, that you smell good? Do you immediately want to sniff your armpits, worrying that the person is being ironic or making fun of you? Or do you simply smile and say, "Chanel No. 5 says thank you!" Being able to see the lighter side of an awkward situation and having the ability to laugh at oneself is paramount to survival in this sometimes harsh and often rude society we live in.

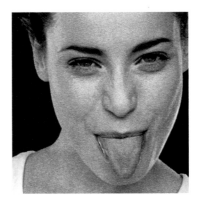

Yuliya Malamud

Humor also has a strong tie to optimism. *Optimism* is defined as "an inclination to put the most favorable construction upon actions and events, or to anticipate the best possible outcome." In other words, combined with humor, optimism allows you to think the best of people instead of the worst. When that stranger says you smell good, as an optimist, you have to smile to yourself and think, "Well, I'm glad I took a bath today." When you have no sense of humor and are a pessimist, you instead wonder, "Who is that pervert and why is he smelling me?" It's no big deal. Don't get offended. Now, if some stranger tells you that you have a "nice ass" (instead of saying, "What a lovely pair of jeans"), then, sure, you have reason to get a bit distressed. But instead of reacting in anger, how about laughing it off and replying, as you walk away, "My mama always taught me to shake my moneymaker!" With the number of rude and inappropriate people you are going to randomly encounter in your lifetime, it just isn't worth the time or energy it takes to get upset.

Beginning models often have no formal training in how to walk in the six-inch heels that they frequently are required to wear. I've tried it myself, so I know it's extremely difficult. Yet professional models eventually need to walk in their stilettos like they were born in them. On *ANTM*, the unparalleled runway expert Miss J. Alexander is usually close at hand, however, to coach new girls in the art. He is very vocal and is not afraid to poke fun with some seemingly off-color comments. But his criticism is actually filled with humor, with the intent of getting his "students" to take themselves less seriously. Those who "get it" open up and improve. Those who don't shrink like violets in a hothouse. How would you react to Miss J.'s following barbs?

"My motto is, walk like it's for sale and the rent is due tonight."

"OK, girls, so that was your first fashion experience, and personally I think you all sucked."

"Girl, you walk like you're on crack. Your eyes are so bugged out of your head, like something just scared the hell out of you."

"Your walk was as useless as a flashlight with no batteries in the dark."

"You walk like you're chewin' gum between your legs."

"It's not my place to put anyone down. I am put here to build their egos up. I feel for the models [when they] trip or flub up, and I try hard to contain my laughter. But, child . . . sometimes I just gotta laugh."
        —Miss J. Alexander

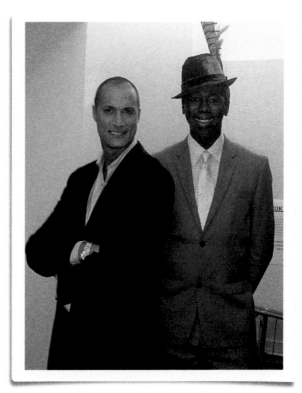

With Miss J. Alexander

MAKE 'EM LAUGH

The American Film Institute compiles lists of America's best and most enduring movies, selected by a blue-ribbon panel of leaders from across the film community. Check out the institute's top-ten-ranked comedy films of all time, from the list "AFI's 100 Years . . . 100 Laughs."

1. *Some Like It Hot* (1959)
2. *Tootsie* (1982)
3. *Dr. Strangelove or: How I Learned to Stop Worrying and Love the Bomb* (1964)
4. *Annie Hall* (1977)
5. *Duck Soup* (1933)
6. *Blazing Saddles* (1974)
7. *MASH* (1970)
8. *It Happened One Night* (1934)
9. *The Graduate* (1967)
10. *Airplane!* (1980)

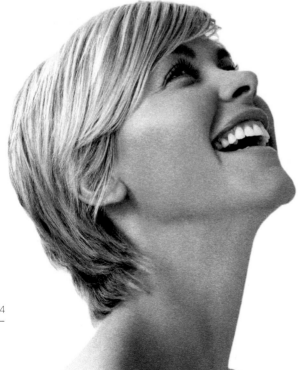

Why do people spend their hard-earned money and suffer long lines to see stand-up, sketch comedy, and funny movies? Because they want to laugh, of course. Laughter is the best medicine, and you don't need a prescription from a doctor, because all these remedies are over the counter! And when you go out to a club or movie theater, you put yourself in good company, among others who are also in need of a laugh. But beware—laughter is contagious. Far more so than the common cold.

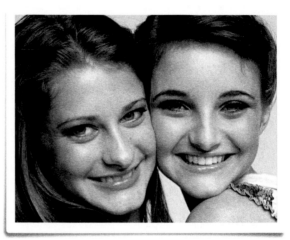

Nicole Ray Muller (right) with her sister, Andrea Muller

Sharing laughs unites people. It is also clinically proven to improve health. Humor is strong medicine for stress, conflict, pain, and depression. A good long laugh can relax your whole body as well as (if not better than) a dip in the Jacuzzi or a massage. Laughing actually boosts your immune system and causes the release of endorphins, the body's natural feel-good chemicals.

When you're exposed to something hilarious in a group situation, an epidemic of those feel-good vibes breaks out. The results are spontaneity, a release of inhibitions, joy, and a lack of defensiveness. Not a bad set of symptoms. So it's no wonder we pay to laugh. It's also no wonder that we are drawn to people who are funny. It's the natural cure for what ails you.

Rachel Cyriacks

LAUGHTER IS THE BEST MEDICINE

According to www.helpguide.org, a nonprofit resource for helping "understand, prevent, and resolve life's challenges," here are the benefits of laughter:

PHYSICAL-HEALTH BENEFITS

- Boosts immunity
- Decreases stress hormones
- Decreases pain
- Relaxes your muscles
- Helps prevent heart disease

MENTAL-HEALTH BENEFITS

- Adds joy and zest to life
- Eases anxiety and fear
- Relieves stress
- Improves mood
- Enhances resilience

SOCIAL BENEFITS

- Strengthens relationships
- Attracts others to us
- Enhances teamwork
- Helps defuse conflict
- Promotes group bonding

THE LAUGH TRACK

Of course, too much of a good thing can be wicked bad. It's annoying when you meet someone who laughs at every single thing. While humor and laughter are vital to our equation, so is balance. People who don't seem to take anything seriously can really become tiresome.

Personally, I am often wary of people who laugh at everything I say, as if the words that come out of my mouth all amount to a joke—especially in professional situations. Or worse yet, people who find themselves hysterical and burst into peals of laughter after every *blah, blah, blah* they speak. I often feel like shouting out to these people, "Dial it down a notch!"

It makes me wonder, too, what is truly behind that person's incessant laugh. Is it that they think it's a form of flattery to find me the funniest person on earth since Lucille Ball? Do they want something from me? Are they trying (too hard!) to get me to like them? Or are they just nervous and painfully insecure, laughing everything away to cover up the fact that they are scared to death? More often than not, fortunately, I've found that this maddening behavior stems from insecurity, from the person radiating their discomfort, and that they usually calm down once they realize they are in a safe environment.

In the inimitable words of Steve Martin, "Comedy is the art of making people laugh without making them puke."

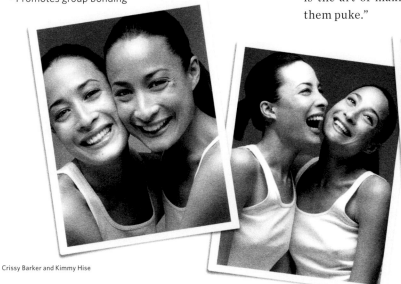

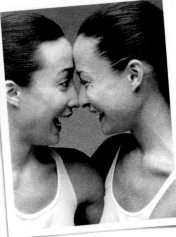

Crissy Barker and Kimmy Hise

PUT A LID ON IT

"Laughter equals pain plus time."
—Comedian Lenny Bruce

Laughing at someone is not nearly the same thing as laughing with someone. In fact, one of the key elements to possessing a good sense of humor is having the common sense to know when something's *not* funny. Even if you really think something is a knee-slapper, will it embarrass someone else if you cackle? Think about it. Maybe now is not the time. Some things become funny in retrospect and, like a fine wine, require some time to pass before the laughter is ready to pour.

As soon as you make someone the butt of your joke, especially an easy target, you run the risk of really hurting someone's feelings. When this happens, your Beauty Equation most definitely will fall like an overcooked soufflé. In theory, it sounds simple enough: Remember to laugh at yourself and not to laugh at others. But obviously, life is a bit more complicated than that, and sometimes we just can't help ourselves. It is very easy to be caught with your guard down and spontaneously erupt in laughter when it's inappropriate. And although a laugh at someone else's expense might be difficult or uncomfortable to stifle, it's always the wisest option if you're at all able.

It boils down to being sensitive to your environment and the people you share it with. Pay attention! Most of us have the tendency to focus on ourselves and what's happening in our own lives. It's easy to half listen to others or zone out. How often do you find yourself "tuning in" halfway through a friend's story? Or what about drifting off in your mind while someone is talking and then having to cover for it? Do you sometimes find yourself laughing at a friend's story, and then suddenly realize you have no idea what it was about, because you were going over the shopping list in your head or thinking about what your boyfriend said on the phone yesterday? Not a pretty situation. Especially if someone is telling you something of a sensitive nature. What kind of friend are you if you are completely unaware of mortifying someone with a total lack of understanding?

SAY CHEESE!

One of the hardest things to capture on camera is a natural-looking smile or laugh. Shouting "Smile" or telling your subject "This is a smile shot" never has the desired effect. And forget about "Say cheese," unless, of course, it's said with enough irony to elicit a wry laugh. Sure, when you ask your subject to show their pearly whites, their face might imitate a smile or laugh on demand, but 99 percent of the time, their eyes tell a completely different story. It's one of the reasons I chat with my models so much when trying to get a candid shot, because when you can catch someone off guard, perhaps even in the middle of a real giggle, that's when the real magic happens.

People are often uncomfortable having a good belly laugh in front of the camera, scared that they will be caught looking crazy, mouth wide open or even drooling or something! Sure, you might not look all that becoming at the climax, but just before and just after, you'll look sublime.

Funny thing is, this also translates outside the photo studio. You go to a party or an event where you are surrounded by people you don't know, and instead of being your naturally gorgeous self and appearing comfortable, with a light smile and look of ease in your eyes, you might find yourself trying to appear cool, or tough and sophisticated. The truth is, though, instead of being noticed around the room as beautiful, you might come off as pompous, boring, or rude. It's a protection mechanism that we all too often fall prey to, but it invariably backfires.

ANTM contestant Fatima Siad, revealing her beautifully natural smile

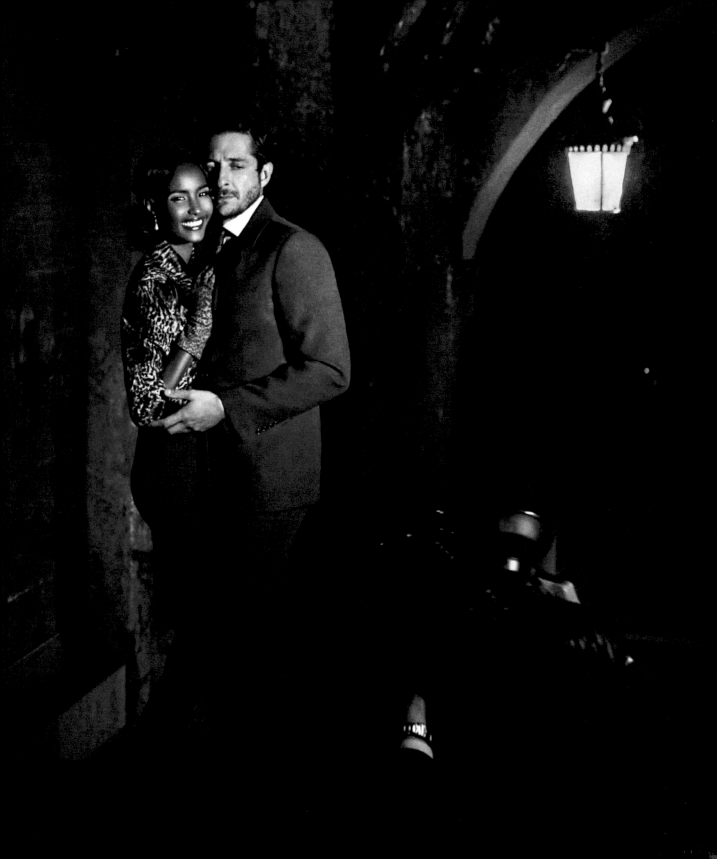

"Button up your shirt. It's not sexy. It's animal." —*Beverly Hills Cop* **(1984)**

I have often noticed that when an A-list celebrity walks into a room, they usually seem like they can socialize confidently with everyone, while their entourage betrays them, never removing their sunglasses or hats and barely talking to one another, let alone mingling. If this is how their friends behave, imagine what these people must be like when the cameras aren't rolling or the crowd isn't watching. Boring! Not sexy, not pretty, and certainly not beautiful. Realize that we all potentially have that star quality, and it's called having a sense a humor. Don't take yourself so seriously that you think a grin won't look good. A smile never goes out of vogue, and should be something you always wear out, unless you're going to a funeral.

Conversely, quite often, when you're the one who's always cracking jokes, playing the fool, or being the court jester, it's because you're hiding a deeper insecurity. And although it's admirable to put on a brave face and have a sense of humor, it's not healthy to avoid reality or be in denial.

It's so easy to believe that the world revolves around you, and in some ways it does. Your little universe is exactly that—but we need to remember that we all sort of feel that way. It's hard to think of anything more annoying than meeting someone who believes their life is more important than yours or who's completely oblivious to the rest of the world because they are so wrapped up in themselves. People in fashion and entertainment suffer from this affliction in rather high numbers. Partly because they mistakenly think they are in the know and too cool for school. And partly because, sadly, we hero-worship them.

MODEL ZINGERS

Funny, not so funny right now, or over-the-top? You decide!

KORTNIE COLE, *ANTM*
"My body is a temple, and my temple wants cheesecake."

CINDY CRAWFORD, supermodel
"Even I don't wake up looking like Cindy Crawford."

CHRISTIE TURLINGTON, supermodel
"I think if my butt's not too big for them to be photographing it, then it shouldn't be too big for me."

TIFFANY RICHARDSON, *ANTM*
"That skank ho poured beer on my weave! It's not even my hair!"

JANICE DICKINSON, supermodel
"If you think I'm over the top, I am!"

(**D O W N L O A D**)

SONGS ABOUT... LAUGHING MATTERS BY FUNNY PEOPLE

"I wore a see-through dress and nobody looked!"

....

"Satisfaction (I Can't Get No)" —PHYLLIS DILLER

"Twisted" —BETTE MIDLER

"Rappin' Rodney" —RODNEY DANGERFIELD

"King Tut" —STEVE MARTIN

"The Chanukah Song" —ADAM SANDLER

"Nigel and I have an amazing crew of people who we work, create, and, most importantly, laugh with. There are projects that require that we travel to all corners of the globe and shoot into the wee hours of the morning. Being in a state of 'humor' is the magic that brings people together and produces the best work."

—Crissy Barker

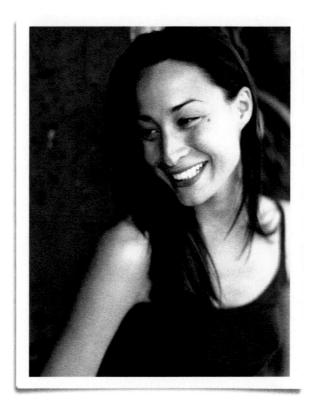

A FINAL WORD—THE LAST LAUGH

"Comedy is simply a funny way of being serious," said dramatic actor Peter Ustinov. Or as my grandma would say, "There is much truth in jest, child!"

Whenever you're critiqued, it's easy to take offense. It's far wiser, though, to take it with a light heart and laugh. Still, understand that there can be a lot of truth in comic banter. You've heard the expression "Live and learn," haven't you? Well, I like to say, "Laugh and learn."

Humor is the common denominator of life. It helps us get to the root of the most complex of issues—our own included. The funniest comedians reveal patterns of human nature that are so true they make us laugh in recognition. Turn that power onto your own life and you will find yourself growing in ways you never imagined possible. You only have one life to live, so make sure to have the last laugh.

Comedy Hour: *the challenge*

1. FUNNY FACE

Do you have any funny props lying around? Perhaps a pair of big glasses with a false nose and a moustache? A multicolored wig? A pair of wax lips? For this exercise, I want you to crack yourself up. Put on something ridiculous and show the camera you can laugh at yourself and not take things so seriously. Take a self-portrait!

2. A LAUGHING MATTER

Take your camera with you today wherever you go. The goal here is to try and capture others in a laugh. How will you do it? The technique is up to you. But in the end, you will select a photo, whether of your father, partner, friend, coworker, or total stranger, in the act of being happy and laughing.

3. I'VE RUN OUT OF IDEAS!

That's it. I have no more tips or ideas, so . . . maybe just snap a quick self-portrait? PS: That was a joke. Did it make you laugh? Seriously, ladies and germs (Did I use that joke already? Told you I was out of ideas!), I do want you to take another self-portrait, but guess what? This one you are going to have to invent by yourself. I'm sure you've had a brilliant photo idea of your own while doing all of our challenges. Now's your chance to show yourself doing your own thing, your way. And I want everyone to share their ideas with all of us at www.beautyequation.com, explaining your inspiration. Take some time to go back through everything we've done together. Reflect on it. Take it all in. Look at your very first portrait (and if that doesn't make you laugh, nothing will!). Close your eyes, think about how much fun you have had and how much you've learned—about yourself, others, me, photography, beauty, all of it. Release yourself from any remaining insecurities; open your eyes. Now set up and take your self-designed self-portrait. I love it already. Do you?

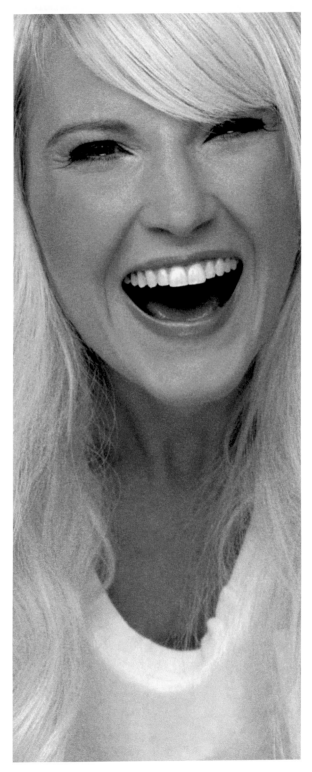

SO remember, use your sense of humor to help balance out the compliments and the criticisms, take rudeness and inappropriateness with a grain of salt, and know that without humor, your health and your sanity are at risk. And no matter how successful you become in your field, keep your feet on the ground, even when they are in six-inch heels! Laugh at yourself rather than at others, and while you're at it, pay attention to others rather than just yourself. Laugh, but listen. Listen, but contribute. Be funny, but don't try to control the room. Smile from your heart, not your head, even if it's spinning from trying to keep all of this straight.

What you're after is displaying a sense of humor in the moment, and the challenge is to be neither ahead of yourself nor behind the curve, but, instead, right on the mark. Divide every element of your Beauty Equation with humor, and you can conquer the essence of all I have put before you in this book. The most beautiful you is someone who smiles, laughs, and is in on the joke of life. It's all a mystery, it's all a process, and the only way to enjoy it fully is to never take it all too seriously.

Alissa Laderer, twenty-five, actress, capturing humor

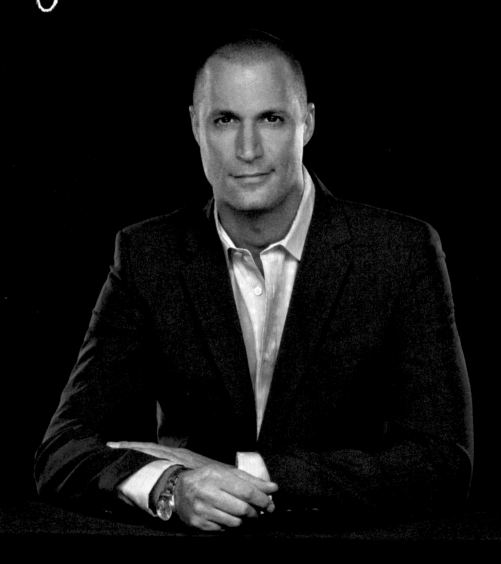

> "Above all, be kind to yourself and allow your true beauty to shine through. Only you can be that beautiful."
> —Nigel Barker

You Be the Judge: *the final teach*

AND THE WINNER IS . . . YOU

Through the course of this book we have captivated ourselves with *allure*, become emboldened with *confidence*, concerned by *compassion*, invigorated with *spontaneity*, gotten the skinny on *radiance*, gotten wise to *health*, been inspired by *honesty*, enamored by *charm*, motivated with *energy*, and tickled by *humor*!

Now it's time to add up all the pieces of the pie, and reveal your Beauty Equation—to yourself. In the end, it doesn't matter what anyone else thinks. There is no panel of judges waiting to tell you what looks good or what feels sexy. There is only you, every day, waking up to yourself, wanting to be the best *you* possible.

1. THE SUM OF YOU

Channeling each chapter in the book, take a few minutes to write an entry encapsulating the definition of your Beauty Equation in your own figurative words. What is your final summation? Try to define what all of the chapters add up to for you. After contemplating what you've written, set up your camera and take a final self-portrait that conveys your formula and your success.

2. "TELL A VISION"

Combining everything you've learned from the *Beauty Equation*, videotape yourself looking straight into the camera, explaining how you feel the book has changed you. Wrap it up with any tips you have for the rest of the world.

ONE LAST FINAL WORD—CURTAIN CALL

It's been a delight sharing the experience I've gained over the past twenty years with you. As a father of two lovely children, there's nothing I want more than for them to grow up striving to be as beautiful as they can, from the inside out, by embracing their own Beauty Equation. It's a gift we can each possess if we're up for the challenge. So, while I hope I have helped you on your path to your own Beauty Equation, remember, you did all the work. Give your beautiful self a well-deserved pat on the back!

The many faces of the *Beauty Equation* (from top, left to right):
Mercedes Andrews, Roselyn Azcona, Lena Marti, Lauren Cotton
Courtney Lavine, Jami Kinton, Rachel Oyama, Nicole Ray Muller, Ruwaida Jawando
Lulu Braithwaite, Alissa Laderer
Yuliya Malamud, Neha Chheda
Shannon Rusbuldt

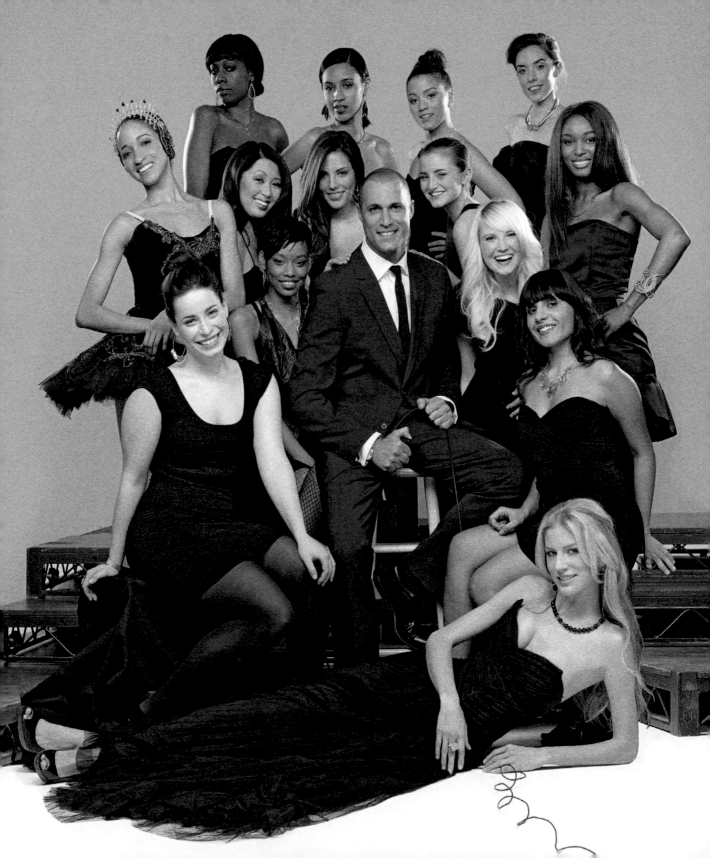

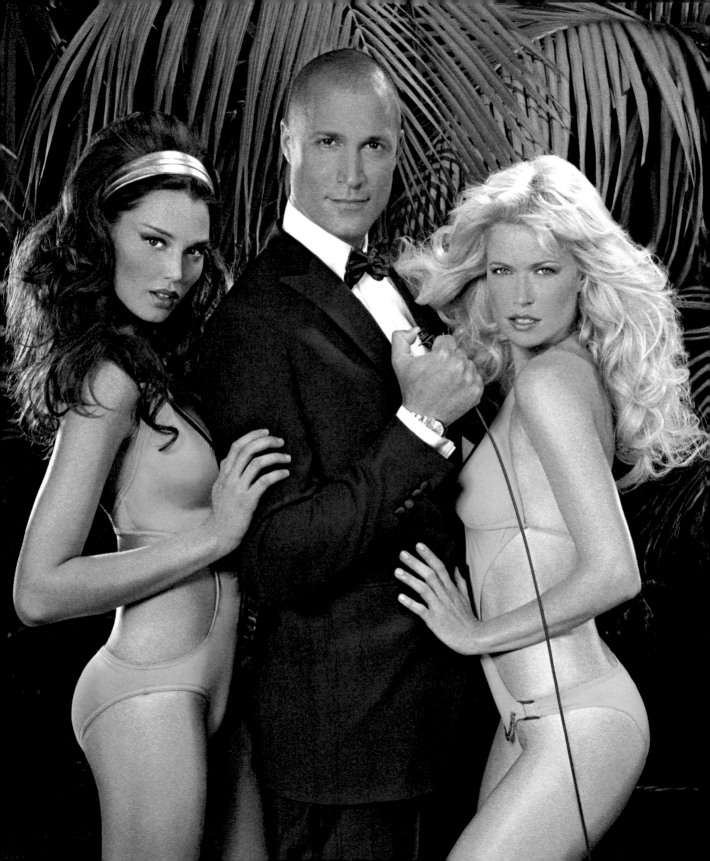

Dr. Photo's Guide to Better Photography

DISCOVERING your Beauty Equation is your goal; the camera is the tool you'll use to help achieve your formula. I'm sure, at this point, pretty much everyone has used a camera of one sort or another. My four-year-old son is already following in my footsteps, constantly running around the studio with his digital camera, taking, deleting, and even downloading photos.

How involved you get technically is entirely your call. As I will outline below, anything goes. Any way you do it, you can make it work. I may be biased, but I think you will find that if you put a little effort into understanding some basic (and fun!) precepts of photography, you will really enjoy taking your pictures one step further. We've all taken a lucky great shot, one that you just snapped and it came out beautifully, but by applying some of my tips, you can take luck out of the equation and perhaps even discover a new hobby.

Dr. Photo, armed with all your photography tips and tricks,
and models Amanda Irby (left) and Melissa Keller

You can use any camera to take your self-portraits and photo assignments for the Beauty Equation. I recommend that you use a device that allows you to easily upload your images at www.beautyequation .com so you can create your own online portfolio.

Of course, you can also use a film camera and scan your prints. And there's no need to go digital either. You can always create an actual physical portfolio/ diary/scrapbook with your picture prints, a pen, and glue. Whatever makes you comfortable.

Anything from the ever-popular and easy-to-use compact point-and-shoot digital cameras to the sophisticated digital SLRs will do the trick. Most of today's camcorders, phones, and computers have both still and video camera options as well. Obviously, some of these devices will deliver bigger images and clearer pictures than others, but that doesn't mean one is better than the next when it comes to the real task at hand. After all, we're not trying to build careers in photography; we're developing your Beauty Equation. Work with what you've got and, through some of my photo tips, I'll do all I can to help you get the best shots possible.

COMPACT DIGITAL CAMERAS (Point-and-shoots)

This is the most popular type of camera for the average user. The lens doesn't come off the camera; everything (including autoexposure and autofocus) is built into a sleek little package that can fit in your purse or pocket. Depending on the price, these cameras come loaded with all sorts of bells and whistles, usually to add fun effects to your pictures. One thing not to get hung up on is the megapixel level of your camera. This can matter when you're blowing your pictures up to billboard size, but for the scale and format we're working in, anything above 2 megapixels will suffice. One necessary distinction you should pay attention to, however, is digital versus optical zoom. Simply put, digital zoom = bad, and optical zoom = good. Digital zooms attempt to mimic what optical zooms do,

but they can't. I suggest you go for the highest optical zoom available—which is currently all the way up to 20x on some consumer cameras—but make sure you have at least 5x to be able to get a good beauty (face) shot. The point is that you want to be able to set the camera up far enough away from yourself that the camera is not functioning at a wide angle, which can make you look distorted.

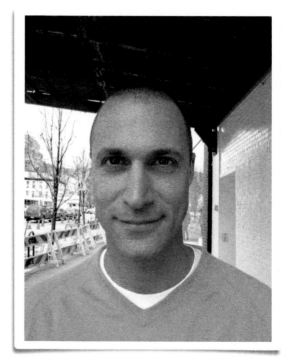

This shot was taken too close to my face. The wide angle of the lens = distortion.

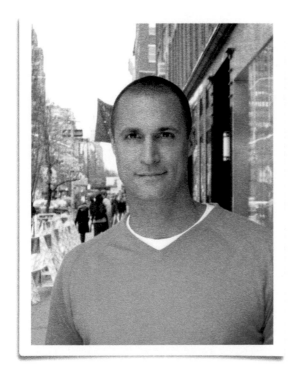
Now, using the optical zoom allows the camera to be far enough away to keep me in proportion. This is the shot you want.

If there is one feature you should find and use on this type of camera, it's the "portrait" mode. "Portrait" mode is perfect for most of our photo assignments. It automatically puts all of the focus on you or whatever you are shooting. How? The rest of the shot, the background, is set so that it will go out of focus in most lighting scenarios, and will usually come out slightly blurry, thus pulling the viewer's eye to you. The proper term for this is *depth of focus* and, for a portrait, the idea is that it keeps all attention on the subject.

Some of the newer cameras have great low-light sensitivity, allowing you to take your portraits at night or inside without a flash, to give a more realistic look. Because we are experimenting with all sorts of different lighting scenarios, you will definitely want to get out your camera manual and find out how to turn off the automatic flash.

A DSLR is a "professional-looking" camera that comes with changeable lenses. It allows you to manually focus and command a lot more control over your images than a compact camera does. It also comes with automatic settings that give you sharper results than their compact cousins. If you choose this type of camera, I encourage you to play. Dare to experiment with the manual settings: aperture, ISO, and lens length.

Most DSLRs will have an "A" or "AV" setting, which stands for aperture. In the simplest of explanations, the word *aperture* is equivalent to *opening*. The more "open" your lens is, the more light it is letting in. Literally, your lens opens wider or smaller. In bright light, the lens doesn't need to be as wide open as it does in darker conditions to get the right amount of light to expose your photo correctly. Think of being in a room with blinds on a sunny morning. With the blinds closed, you can still feel the sun light up the room. Compare that to an overcast day, when it feels like night when it's actually time to go to work. You need to open the blinds completely to compensate for the lack of light.

Aperture works in the same way—the number of your aperture setting is based on the amount of available light and indicates the wideness of the opening. A lower aperture setting is good when the light is low, resulting in your lens being wider open to compensate. In other words, in darker conditions, you will get a light reading of 2.8 or 5.6. In order to keep your shots from being underexposed by the lack of light, the lower setting of your aperture means there will be a bigger hole in the lens (aperture = hole), letting in more light. Conversely, in bright sunlight, you will get a light reading of 16 or 22 and, in order to keep your shots from being overexposed by all that light, the higher setting of your aperture reduces the size of the hole in your lens, thus balancing your exposure.

When you're using an automatic camera, the lens is also doing this, but the camera is deciding for you how open or closed to make the lens and so, of course, it's also deciding what the picture will look like. The area in the frame with the most light will get the "attention" of an automatic camera, whether you like it or not. That's how the table lamp ends up in focus while your face is a blur!

"Hey, Nigel," you throw in. "Why would I give a hoot if my lens is more opened or more closed?" Good question! The answer lies in the look of the picture you are trying to achieve. Again, this is just the simple answer, as there are variables, but bright light and a closed-down lens tends to allow more objects in the frame to be in focus, while lower light and a more open lens lets the focus fall on the object of your choice, while throwing everything else into soft focus. Another thing to consider is that, if you are sitting in a dimly lit part of a room, "opening the lens up" keeps you from underexposing your face, even if the background then ends up overexposed; if you are

under the bright sun, "closing the lens down" keeps you from overexposing your face, even if the shaded background then goes completely dark. In other words, manually adjusting the aperture lets you choose which level of light in which part of the frame you want to focus on.

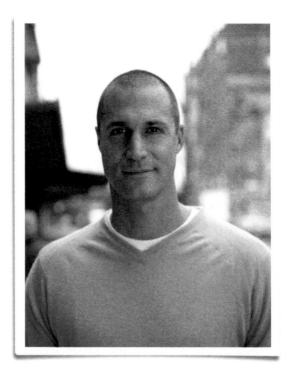

Now, this shot is taken using a low aperture, creating a shallow depth of field. Notice how I'm in focus and the background is blurred. This makes for a better portrait.

A warning: If you are in "A" or "AV" mode, and you set your aperture to a low setting, between 2.8 and 5.6, the shutter speed will automatically change to compensate for any light reading. In general, that's a good thing. It means the lens will remain open long enough to expose the picture properly. But here's the rub: The longer it takes for the shutter to open and close, the easier it is for the picture to go out of focus. When you set the aperture to 2.8 in a low-light situation, the shutter *o-pens ver-y slow-ly, holllllds o-pen, then fi-nal-ly clos-es* . . . almost like it is in slow motion. If the camera moves at all, you are guaranteed a blurry shot. And even if the camera is locked down on a tripod, slight movements of your face or body in

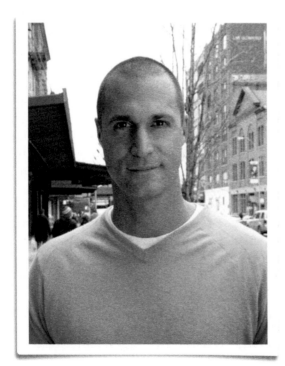

This shot is taken using a high aperture, creating a long depth of field. I'm in focus, but so is the background, which is a little distracting.

200

front of a slow-moving shutter will cause the image to lose focus too.

So now what? In your self-portraits, you want to manually set your aperture to a low setting to concentrate the focus on you. And by increasing something called your ISO, you will increase your shutter speed, so you will still be able to take dynamic shots, even in low light.

"Uh, Nigel? What's my ISO?" Another good question! ISO denotes how sensitive the image sensor is to the amount of light present. "Huh?" Here's a simple equation to remember: High ISO = better for low light. The higher the ISO, the more sensitive the image sensor, and therefore you increase your ability to take pictures in dimly lit situations. I recommend changing the ISO to 400 or higher, so the shutter speed will automatically increase, thus reducing blurring of your facial movements. There is a price to pay, though, and you'll have to judge for yourself if you like it: The higher the ISO, the more "noisy" your pictures get, which means they can look "grainy." You could say that was "bad," but sometimes clients pay me a lot of money to give them that look. All of these choices are a matter of taste, which is why I encourage you to play with your settings. Take the exact same photo five different times with different aperture and ISO settings, and compare them to see what you prefer.

Now for lenses. In general, I recommend using a lens length of 50 to 105mm. Anywhere in that range will be fine, but the closer to 50mm you go, the wider the picture, which isn't great for a close-up portrait. It may seem backward, but the "tighter" lens literally "widens" the image. (You've seen "fish-eye" photos, right? Those are from extremely wide lenses.) Longer lenses, closer to 105mm, on the other hand, compact the image (thus making beauty shots more beautiful), but you'll have farther to run after you press the self-timer! Now you see why they are called "longer" lenses. The distance to subject is the part that is "longer," not the actual lens. Another tip: The closer the lens size is to 105mm, the less distortion you'll see in your close-up photos and the prettier the picture will be—think of it as tightening your pores for you.

VIDEO CAMERAS

In the *Beauty Equation,* there are a number of fun challenges that will require a camera that can capture video. Most digital "still" cameras now come with this ability (conversely, many video cameras, even older ones, come with the ability to capture still images). Get out those manuals and figure it out! Tip: If you run an Internet search using your camera's model number and brand name plus the word *manual,* you can probably find an online version.

When shooting yourself in motion, again, I recommend sitting a little farther away from your video camera and zooming in to achieve a close-up crop on the picture. And if you get a camera where you can flip the video-monitor screen around, when you go to sit down in position for your shot, you can see yourself and the crop.

Video cameras also have manual settings, and the exact same rules apply as with a still camera. One thing about video to bear in mind, though, is that it has a much harder time dealing with large differences in light. You know how you can't get your video camera to focus on Aunt Jane's face when there's a window in the frame? Or how after that family picnic, all you could see of your favorite cousins were fuzzy images, even though the sunny picnic table in the back was in perfect focus? That's why! Again, using your manual settings can help balance that out, but whereas a still camera will create interesting effects with differences in light intensity, video just freaks out. So whether you decide to wrap your head around all of the manual stuff or prefer to stick with the automatic settings on a point-and-shoot camcorder, try to seek out even lighting situations when you do your video challenges. If you're outside, sit either in direct light with no shade in sight, or in the shade—making sure there isn't some object way behind you reflecting the blazing sun. Also, if you are in direct sunlight, don't sit so that you have to squint into the camera. Treat the sun like a lightbulb and "place" yourself where the sun shines on you to the most flattering effect. If you're inside, don't frame yourself in a shot that contains an exposed bulb, avoid sitting by windows, and look for a spot near the brightest light in the room. And while you're at it, check out the background—is there anything there that will flare or attract light and ruin your frame, like a stainless steel refrigerator or a mirror?

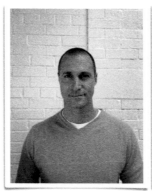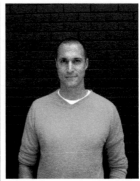

In this shot, the bright white background has created a "backlit" effect. Because the background is so bright, the camera phone delivers an underexposed image. (Notice how dark I am.)

Now, this shot is taken with the same lighting, but a darker background. The camera phone automatically adjusts the light reading, producing a better overall exposure.

And no matter what camera you are using, remember, lighting is still lighting. You can use the cheapest camera phone in existence and improve the image dramatically by understanding the basic concepts of illumination and by using the three-point lighting tips outlined in the sidebar on page 204.

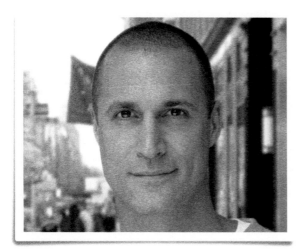

This shot is taken with a camcorder. Notice how evenly exposed the portrait is. By positioning myself in the same lighting as my background, I was able to capture an image without any conflicting light sources. (This may have also caused me to be out of focus.)

CAMERA PHONES

Although they're not my first choice, camera phones, used carefully, can actually result in more-than-decent photos. Most camera phones also now come equipped with video capture and are easy to download to your computer, so you'll be all set with one gadget.

Usually, camera phones take an overall light reading of the whole frame before firing. The rules, then, are very similar to video. You want to avoid being "backlit." If you are standing in front of a window in daylight, the background is brighter than the foreground, so your face will come out dark, sometimes to the point of looking like a silhouette. If the light on you is very bright and the background is dark, the object you want to focus on could end up looking overexposed. So look for places where the light is even. For example, a place in the shade where you can stand up against a wall. If you need additional light to expose the shot correctly, make sure the lamp or light you are using is aimed at your face at head level. That way your eyes will be lit up instead of becoming dark holes.

BUILT-IN COMPUTER CAMERAS AND WEB CAMERAS

Cameras that come built in to your computer or external Web cameras that connect directly to your computer work well, because you can check out the light and framing as you go. You can even use the light from your screen to help illuminate yourself. The tip here is to make sure that your computer is at a higher angle than you are. If you have it on your desk and you are looking down at the screen, the results can be unflattering and give you "ghoul lighting." Either scoot down lower or prop your laptop up on a stack of books so that your head is at the same position as the camera at the top of the screen.

These cameras also allow you to capture video. If your computer didn't come with a built-in camera, adding a Web cam will cost about a quarter of the price of a real camera, so if you're on a budget, it could be a great option.

Also, often the light we use at our desks has nothing to do with looking at ourselves. We're busy looking at what we're reading or drawing or editing, not worrying about what our faces look like. If you are going to do the bulk of the Beauty Equation challenges at your computer station, set up a simple lighting scenario using some of the tips here. A bonus: With even a little attention to lighting, your friends will start complimenting you on how great you look during video chat sessions.

While we are on the subject, here's a little secret I've discovered. When using your computer/Web camera for taking a photo, video, or for video chatting, make the desktop background on your computer a totally blank white field. When you do this, your computer screen acts as a "soft box," a device for creating diffused lighting that I often employ for an even, flattering effect. Try it!

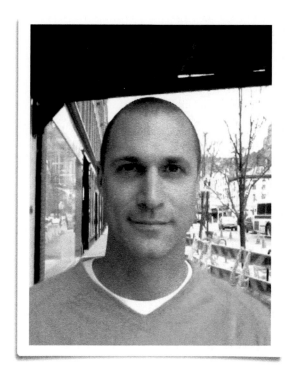

This shot is taken with my laptop. By holding the laptop slightly above me, I was able to position myself directly in front of the camera and capture a workable portrait.

THREE THINGS TO THINK ABOUT WITH ANY KIND OF LIGHTING

All lighting combines three key elements: direction, intensity, and quality. When setting up a shot, if you think about using them to bring out the feeling you hope to create, you will add to the overall success of every challenge. Remember, there is no right answer when it comes to lighting, only a desired effect and understanding how to achieve it.

1. DIRECTION: Where is the light that is hitting your subject coming from? From the side, the back, the top, below, or all of the above? Think about the sun. What direction is it hitting your face from, and how will it be different at another time of day? Look at a horror photo of a monster. Bet you the light is coming from underneath, an unnatural direction often associated with evil.

2. INTENSITY: How bright is the light on your subject? If you are setting up lights and they feel too bright, back them away from the subject. Not enough light for you? Add more lamps or move the ones you have closer. Do you want one side of the face to be lit more intensely than the other, like an emotionally conflicted film-noir heroine? Or do you want to look evenly lit, like a girl next door?

3. QUALITY: How would you describe the feeling of the light you want in color and in mood? Clear white lights, like fluorescents, feel cold. Amber lights, like candles, feel warm. Light pointed directly at your subject, like the sun when it isn't behind clouds, feels hard. Indirect light, like light that bounces off the walls or comes filtered through curtains, feels soft. If the effect you want to achieve is "romance," and you would describe that as "soft and warm," what could you do to alter the quality of your bedroom light to give that feeling?

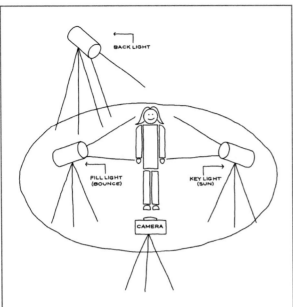

BACK LIGHT

FILL LIGHT
(BOUNCE)

KEY LIGHT
(SUN)

CAMERA

THREE-POINT LIGHTING

Three-point lighting is the basis of all studio photography and film shoots, and it is exactly what it sounds like: lighting from three different places.

Your *key light* sits off-center from the camera and provides the main source of light to your face. In a "natural light" setup, it might be the place where the sunlight enters the room. In a lighting setup, it is the strongest source of light, aimed toward one side of your face.

Your *fill light* balances out the other side of your face, literally filling in the darkness and shadows caused by the key light. If you want an even look, your fill light and your key light will be of similar intensity. If you want a more dramatic look, your fill light will be either of lower wattage, farther away, or even non-existent. Ever see photographers out in the street and there's some crazy-looking dude balancing a reflector that's pointed at the model? The photographer is probably using the sun as her key light and the dude is trying to intensify it; or conversely, the sun is so bright from one direction that they are trying to bounce it onto the other side of the face and increase their fill. Suddenly makes a lot of sense, right?

The last light in the equation is your *back light* (aka hair/shoulder light). It tends not to be as strong, and you use it to separate yourself from the background, to give that little bit of glow to your hair and/or body.

TIPS AND TRICKS

USING SOFT, EVEN LIGHTING

Most people consider this type of lighting to be flattering and, I would say, this is the easiest way to achieve "pretty-looking" photos. No matter what kind of camera you are shooting with, find a shady place or room filled with natural light. You don't want the sun to be pouring through the windows; rather, you want the sun to be hidden or behind you. I am not talking about being backlit, either. The light should be indirectly filling the space you're in. This sort of light is soft and gentle. It will not highlight your blemishes or wrinkles, and your eyes will look alive with color. To avoid exposure problems, always make sure that whatever's behind you is lit in the same manner you are.

USING HARDER, MOODIER LIGHTING

Looking for a bit more edge to tell your story? Set up a scenario where you are closer to the light source. Whether the source is a window or a lamp, moving closer will create more drama and shadows and will actually give you more definition and tone in your shots.

LIGHTING WITH A FLASH

You can create many different effects using your on-camera flash. If you are a good distance from your camera, you can use "fill flash" to punch in just enough light that you are exposed to the same degree your background is, maintaining the ambiance in the room, yet lighting your eyes so we don't lose the most important factor of the shot—you! This also works for rendering realistic sunsets.

For an entirely different effect, try this fun trick: Get really close to your camera and turn your flash up high to create that washed-out, old-school-fashion look reminiscent of glamour shots of the fifties. The flash bleaches out all imperfections while lending a dramatic Hollywood feel. This works especially well if you have plenty of makeup on and are already in a well-lit situation.

WHITE BALANCE

Almost every camera lets you adjust the "white balance." What does that mean? Very simply, it means telling the camera what color "white" is in the frame, so that it knows what all the other colors are in relation to it. You might think white is white, but go to any paint store and you will see that "white" comes in many shades with many tints. In fact, look around a white room and, depending on where the light hits the wall, you'll see that it appears to be a range of different colors from gray to beige. Automatic settings on most cameras will seek out the whitest thing in the frame and set to that, but to achieve true white balance, go to your manual settings after you've finished lighting. Tape up a sheet of pure white paper where you will be sitting for your portrait—all you need is a sheet from your computer printer—and manually set the white balance while focused on it.

USING YOUR LENS TO YOUR ADVANTAGE

When you get really close to the mirror to look at, say, something stuck in your eye, do you ever stop to look at the rest of your face from that perspective? Well go to your mirror and have a look; you'll notice that your lateral vision doesn't allow you to see your whole face when you're that close. The same problem occurs with cameras. So many point-and-shoots come with extremely wide lenses—which is great for taking group shots at a party from three feet away. It gets everyone in the frame, but they also probably appear disfigured or not in proportion. No wonder people hate what they look like in those pictures! Now, step away from the mirror, but hold your gaze there. You can see your reflection from head to toe with just a slight glance up and down. With your camera, you can create the same effect by backing up the camera and then zooming in to the shot (extending your lens), thereby eliminating any distortion. Also, if you put your flash on from this farther-back position, you can add that perfect amount of fill flash.

TAKING A SELF-PORTRAIT

Most cameras will give you a ten-second countdown for you to run in front of the lens and compose your shot before it takes the picture. Obviously, with digital cameras you can keep trying until you get it right, but there are also several tips that can help you get it right faster. One of the biggest problems people have with self-timers is that they set up the shot, then hit the shutter release, and the camera moves. Let's start, then, with securing the camera. For just a few dollars, you can buy a mini-tripod that stands less than six inches tall and sits on a desktop. Failing that, I have tried everything from wedging my camera in Play-Doh to sticking it in my shoe with the back of the heel keeping the angle of the lens straight. Whatever your method, remember to press the shutter gently and walk normally to your mark. A simple solution is to place the camera in front of a mirror (either on your vanity table or in the bathroom), and then on some books so that it's at the same height as your neck. When you set up your shot and run back to get in position, not only will you be able to check your look in the mirror, but you will be able to see the crop of the shot in the reflection of the mirror (from the back of your camera)—genius, no?

If using a DSLR, a good, inexpensive investment is a long shutter-release cord. This item allows you to sit down in place and get basically settled, then trigger the autotimer from your chair. You have a full ten seconds before the shutter snaps to relax and strike a pose.

When using a cell phone to take a self-portrait, obviously you have certain restraints, like the length of your arm. I say, just go with it. The photo may not be the best-constructed picture ever, but what we are after is the essence of you, not whether you know how to take a great photograph. By the way, I take photos of myself with my kids and friends all the time by holding the camera and pointing back on myself candidly. It has a certain look . . . maybe not the most flattering look, but, hey, it has a look!

ACKNOWLEDGMENTS

I owe a huge debt of gratitude to the folks at Abrams, especially my editor and friend Deborah Aaronson, art director Michelle Ishay, marketing manager Kerry Liebling, and publicist Claire Bamundo. Thanks also to designer Rodrigo Corral and copy editor Carrie Hornbeck.

I would also like to give a special thanks to Marcus Brooks, who has worked tirelessly by my side for the best part of a decade, helping me cajole a smile from the most unlikely of subjects. To Ali Azios for keeping me on track and on time, even when buried deep in paper. To James Freni for his diligence and hard work. And to Todd Hughes and P. David Ebersole, for helping to make sense of my scribbling and rambling, even when miles away.

A big thanks to Rodney E. Hall and David Tibolla, who have been dressing and making up my models for more than ten years. Also for all the styling, grooming, and artwork of Caroline Blanchard, Eloise Cheung, Allie Lawsen, Dana Bar, and Mindy Saad.

For the much-appreciated photographic assistance of Walter Sassard, Robert Massman, and Maria Karas, and the video brilliance of Francisco Aliwalas and Brian Padden.

To my management team at DMA, Sam Sohaili, Aaron Spiewak, Marc Beckman, and Caitlin Smyth for their continued support.

A special thanks to my *ANTM* family: Tyra Banks, Ken Mok, Miss J. Alexander, Jay Manuel, Dana Gabrion, and Cher Aguilar. And to the truly beautiful contestants in the book, who helped out so eagerly.

To the women, from my granny, who was beautifully wise and eloquent, and my mother, who taught me to be a realistic dreamer, to my sisters, Mary-Anne and Linda-Jane, whose love has never faltered.

And finally, to my divine wife, Crissy, and our children, Jack and Jasmine, who make every day a beautiful one.

Library of Congress Cataloging-in-Publication Data

Barker, Nigel, 1972-
  Nigel Barker's beauty equation : revealing a better and more beautiful you.
    p. cm.
  ISBN 978-0-8109-9642-7 (alk. paper)
  1. Beauty, Personal. I. Title.
  HQ1219.B27 2010
  646.7′042–dc22

                        2010020925

Printed and bound in the United States
10 9 8 7 6 5 4 3 2 1

Abrams Image books are available at special discounts when purchased in quantity for premiums and promotions as well as fundraising or educational use. Special editions can also be created to specification. For details, contact specialmarkets@abramsbooks.com, or the address below.

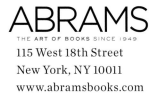

THE ART OF BOOKS SINCE 1949
115 West 18th Street
New York, NY 10011
www.abramsbooks.com

CREDITS: Images courtesy POTTLE PRODUCTIONS, INC. pages 28, 36 (upper left), 74, 91, 128 (left), 134, 158, and 187; Courtesy Sony Entertainment Television pages 84, 85, and 86; Courtesy Richard Dawson Photography pages 124 and 170.